Dramane SOGOBA
Issa KONATE
Sounkalo DAO

# Electrolyte Disorders in a Group of Hospitalized Patients

Dramane SOGOBA
Issa KONATE
Sounkalo DAO

# Electrolyte Disorders in a Group of Hospitalized Patients

## Electrolyte disorders in HIV/AIDS patients in a hospital setting in Bamako, Mali

ScienciaScripts

Cover image: www.ingimage.com

This book is a translation from the original published under ISBN 978-620-6-72197-0.

Publisher:
Sciencia Scripts
is a trademark of
Dodo Books Indian Ocean Ltd. and OmniScriptum S.R.L publishing group

120 High Road, East Finchley, London, N2 9ED, United Kingdom
Str. Armeneasca 28/1, office 1, Chisinau MD-2012, Republic of Moldova, Europe
Printed at: see last page
**ISBN: 978-620-8-19854-1**

Contents

## INTRODUCTION

Infection with the human immunodeficiency virus (HIV), through the immune deficiency it induces, is the cause of various opportunistic infectious complications and cancers. There is an average asymptomatic period of 08 years between infection and the onset of clinical manifestations of the disease, known as acquired immunodeficiency syndrome (AIDS) [1].

At the stage of clinical disease, all the organs are infected by the virus, leading to a number of symptoms, including kidney damage. This affects 10-20% of infected patients and can occur at any stage of HIV infection [2,3].

The clinical presentation of AIDS has changed significantly over the past decade, mainly due to the widespread availability and effectiveness of combination antiretroviral regimens.

Fortunately, the severe complications associated with profound immunodepression are rare in patients who have access to adequate care and treatment. Currently, the most common complications seen in HIV-infected patients are severe but non-AIDS-classifying conditions. These are frequently due to chronic inflammation promoted by the virus itself, and subsequently aggravated by the use of antiretroviral drugs [4, 5, 6].

Renal disorders have been increasingly reported in the context of HIV infection, particularly in addition to decreased glomerular filtration rate (GFR), nephrotic syndrome and proximal tubular failure associated with the use of tenofovir and protease inhibitors such as lopinavir/ritonavir and atazanavir [4,7].

Despite the fact that periodic assessment of renal function (plasma creatinine, GFR) and proteinuria are routinely recommended in the management of these patients. There are very few data on electrolyte disorders in the literature [4,8,9].

Approximately 6% of HIV-infected patients need to be referred to a nephrologist. The reasons for this are varied, and in most cases relate to an added complication of the viral infection. However, the reality of nephropathy associated with HIV infection is currently accepted [10].

HIV-infected patients, particularly those in the advanced stages of the disease, can be affected by infectious, autoimmune and oncological diseases. These diseases are associated with clinical manifestations (such as fever, tachypnea, vomiting, diarrhoea, polyuria and delirium) and may require a variety of medical treatments (antiviral therapy, antibiotics, antineoplastic molecules). This combination of medication and digestive problems predisposes them to developing different types of electrolyte disorders [4, 11,12].

Since AIDS was discovered 34 years ago in Mali, what has been done about it? No specific studies have been carried out on electrolyte disorders, even though some of these disorders are just as lethal as other diseases. We therefore thought it would be interesting to analyse electrolyte disorders in HIV-infected patients during hospitalisation.

**Research question:** What is the frequency of electrolyte disorders in HIV-infected patients in Point G hospitals?

**Research hypotheses :**

- There is a relationship between electrolyte disorders and the clinical signs presented by HIV-infected patients.
- There is a relationship between these electrolyte disorders and the factors that promote them.
- These disorders are either under-recognised or under-appreciated.

## THE OBJECTIVES

**1-General objective :**

To describe electrolyte disorders in HIV/AIDS patients hospitalised in the infectious diseases department of the Point "G" University Hospital.

**2-Specific objectives :**

- determining the frequency of electrolyte disorders in patients ;
- describe the clinical signs associated with electrolyte disorders in patients ;
- identify the factors that contribute to electrolyte disorders.

# 1 GENERAL INFORMATION

## I-1-HIV infection

### I-1-1-Definition :

Infection by the virus results in a progressive deterioration of the immune system, leading to immunodeficiency [13,14].

The term AIDS applies to the most advanced stages of HIV infection, defined by the occurrence of one or more of the twenty opportunistic infections or cancers associated with HIV [13,14].

### I-1-2-History :

On 5 June 1981, the Centers for Disease Control in Atlanta reported several cases of a rare form of pneumonia that specifically affected young homosexual men (3 cases had been reported in 1980).

By the end of that year, it was known that the disease causes immunodeficiency and is transmitted by sexual contact and blood. It was also known to affect not only homosexuals, but also injecting drug users (IDUs) and blood transfusion recipients.

In 1982, a number of researchers around the world began to take action as the disease spread beyond American borders. In France, the disease was observed in hemophiliacs who had received blood transfusions, suggesting that the infectious agent was a virus.

The name AIDS was first used by the scientist Bruce Voeller.

In May 1983, in the journal "Science", Jean-Claude Chermann's team at the Institut Pasteur described for the first time the virus responsible for the disease known as "LymphadenopathyAssociated Virus" or LAV (later HIV-1).

In 1984, the antiretroviral activity of AZT was demonstrated. At the same time, the different modes of transmission of the virus were clearly established.

In 1985, a second virus, LAV-2 (later HIV-2), was isolated from a patient from West Africa.

In 1986, the scientific community adopted the name HIV (human immunodeficiency virus). The first AZT therapy became available, but it remained expensive and highly toxic. The United Nations set up its first AIDS programme.

In 1987, the HIV-2 screening test was developed by "Diagnostics Pasteur".

In 1988, the World Health Organisation (WHO) proclaimed 1er December as World AIDS Day.

In 1994, two drugs (3TC and AZT) were combined, proving to be more effective than a single drug. A Franco-American therapeutic trial showed that transmission of the virus from mother to foetus was reduced with the use of AZT [13,15].

**I-1-3-Epidemiology**

**I-1-3-1-Analytical epidemiology**

**I-1-3-1-1-The pathogenic agent :**

To date, there are two main types of HIV called HIV-1 and HIV-2 [13,16].

**I-1-3-1-1-1-Classification :**

HIV-1 and HIV-2 belong to the retrovirus family. This family is subdivided into three subfamilies according to a classification that takes into account pathogenicity criteria and phylogenetic parameters: *Oncoviruses*, *Spumaviruses* and *Lentiviruses* [17].

- *Oncoviruses*: are associated with tumours and leukaemia. HTLV (Human T-cell Leukemia Virus) belongs to this sub-family. A similar virus called STLV (Simian T Leukemia Virus), whose genome is very close to that of the human virus HTLV-1, was isolated from several monkey species [17].
- *Spumaviruses:* have been identified in many mammals, but have no recognised pathogenicity in humans or animals. [17]
- *Lentiviruses*: cytopathogenic, inducing slowly progressing diseases. Only HIV-1 and HIV-2 are pathogenic for humans [17].

**I-1-3-1-1-2-The structure of HIV**

The AIDS virus includes :

*J* a viral envelope consisting of a lipid bilayer and two types of glycoproteins: gp120 and gp41.

The gp41 molecule crosses the lipid bilayer, while the gp120 molecule occupies a more peripheral position: it acts as a viral receptor for the TCD4 membrane molecule of host cells. The viral envelope is derived from the host cell: as a result, it contains some of the host cell's membrane proteins, including MHC molecules.

*J* a viral core or nucleocapsid, which includes a layer of p17 proteins and a deeper layer of p24 proteins.

*J* a genome consisting of two copies of single-stranded RNA associated with two reverse transcriptase molecules (p64) and other enzyme proteins (p10 protease and p32 integrase) [18].

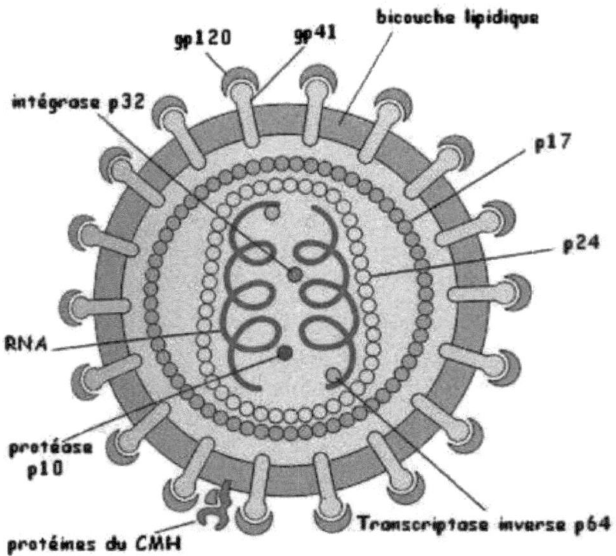

**Figure I: HIV organisational chart** [18].

**I-1-3-1-1-3-Physico-chemical properties :**

HIV is inactivated by most physical and chemical processes used for disinfection or sterilisation [19].

HIV is a heat-sensitive virus. It is inactivated by heating to 56°C for 30 minutes, in less than 15 minutes at a temperature above 100°C (autoclave) [20].

In the external environment, it can survive in aqueous solution for more than 15 days at room temperature (23 to 27°C) and more than 11 days at 37°C.

Its inactivation after drying is complete in 3 to 7 days.

However, this virus is resistant to ionising radiation, whatever the dose used [20].

As for the usual disinfectants, they rapidly inactivate HIV at common concentrations:

Bleach at 12° chlorometric diluted 1:10 inactivates HIV in 15 minutes.

The sensitivity of the virus to sodium hypochlorite means that this disinfectant can be used not only on surfaces, but also to disinfect syringes used by drug addicts.

Aldehydes are highly effective.

Glutaraldehyde at 2% inactivates HIV in 10 minutes, at 0.2% in 30 minutes.

These products are mainly used for disinfecting instruments.

As far as antiseptics are concerned, ethanol (70% alcohol) is active in one minute, polyvidone iodine (Betadine) in 15 minutes, and 2% chlorhexidine

(Hibiscrub, Hibitane), which is not usually very virucidal, is rapidly active here [20].
Quaternary ammonium, an antiseptic and surface disinfectant, inactivates HIV in 10 to 30 minutes at 0.1% [20].
Other chemical agents active on HIV such as: 10% iodine products, phenols, hydrogen peroxide, 0.1% formaldehydes [20].

**I-1-3-1-1-4-Genetic variability** :

While HIV-1 is distributed worldwide, HIV-2 is most prevalent in West Africa.
HIV-1 is divided into three groups:
Group M (main group, >98%),
Group O (outlier, <1%),
Group N (new, <1%).
Group M is responsible for the majority of HIV-1 infections worldwide and can be further subdivided into phylogenetically recognised subtypes (clades): Subtype A: 23%; Subtype B: 8%; Subtype C: 56%; Subtype D: 5%; Subtype E: 5%; and Subtype F-K: 3%. There are also recombinants, which contain a mixture of these subtypes. The most common recombinants are mixtures of subtypes AE and AG; less common are mixtures of subtypes AGHK, AFGHJK, AB, and BC [16].

**I-1-3-1-1-5-The virus reservoir :**

Multiplication of the virus is possible in all mammals, but the reservoir has become strictly human (asymptomatic seropositives and symptomatic patients) [17].
In humans, HIV targets two types of cells: those in which it replicates and those in which it is in a quiescent state.

- Target cells in which HIV replicates: these are cells expressing the CD4 receptor and one of the coreceptors (CCR1, CCR3, CCR5, CCR2b, CXCR4, etc.) on their surface: CD4+ lymphocytes, monocytes and macrophages, dendritic cells, Langherans cells and brain microglial cells [21].
- Target cells in which HIV is quiescent: these are the follicular dendritic cells present in the germinal centres of ganglia [17].

**I-1-3-1-2-Modes of transmission :**

HIV is transmitted in three main ways [22].

**I-1-3-1-2-1-Sexual transmission :**

It is transmitted via the mucous membranes of the mouth, vagina or rectum when they come into contact with sexual secretions or blood containing the virus.

**I-1-3-1-2-2-The homosexual route :**

**It is more** common in the West than in Africa. Given the diversity of sexual practices undertaken by the same individual, seroconversions linked to oral-anal or oral-genital practices between men are rare. However, it is highly probable that a few cases of contamination have occurred [17].

**I-1-3-1-2-3-The heterosexual route :**

It is the most widespread in the world. Worldwide, 75-85% of HIV infections are acquired through unprotected sex, compared with 5-10% among homosexuals [17].

In sub-Saharan Africa and Mali, almost 90% of cases are attributable to heterosexual transmission [17,23].

**I-1-3-1-2-4-Blood transmission :**

It is transmitted via blood containing the virus.

- Transfusion of blood and blood derivatives: improved donor selection and more sensitive screening tests have considerably reduced the risk of contamination by this route [22].
- Intravenous drug use: the practice of sharing needles or products between injecting drug users (IDUs) allows a small quantity of blood to be inoculated venously from one infected person to another. This leads to the transmission of HIV infection [22].
- The reuse of used, non-sterilised needles [17].
- Occupational contamination: transmission among healthcare workers has only been documented in cases of exposure to blood or fluids visibly containing blood. Accidents leading to HIV contamination mainly occurred during wounds or injections with contaminated medical-surgical equipment.

More rarely, it was splashed onto lesioned skin or a mucous membrane. Transmission in the nursing direction is exceptional [17].

African and Malian particularities: traditional practices such as tattooing, scarification, excision, circumcision, etc.

**I-1-3-1-2-5-Vertical or maternal-fctal transmission :**

Transmission of HIV from mother to child can occur at different stages: in utero in the weeks preceding delivery (1/3 of cases), at the time of delivery (2/3 of cases) or during breastfeeding (isolated cases) [17]. The use of ARVs has reduced the rate of HIV transmission by this route by 70%, with only 6% of children affected [24].

**I-1-3-1-2-6-Other modes of transmission :**

Transmission may occur during transplantation. There may be exposure to biological fluids from which HIV has been isolated: saliva, tears, urine, cerebrospinal fluid, bronchoalveolar lavage. But the presence of the virus does not automatically mean that it is transmissible, because of the low concentration of the virus and the possible presence of components that inactivate it. In the case of these biological fluids, the risk of contamination is theoretical, and no case of contamination by HIV through exposure to these fluids without visible blood has been published [22].

**I-1-3-1-3-Factors favouring transmission :**

They depend on the route of transmission.

**I-1-3-1-3-1- Factors favouring sexual transmission :**

- Known HIV-seropositive partner,
- Genital infections or lesions in the partner,
- Sexual intercourse during menstruation,
- Occasional unprotected sex,
- Unprotected anal intercourse,

Microscopic excoriations during sex and genital infections or lesions in the partner are potential entry points for HIV during unprotected sex [17,23].

**I-1-3-1-3-2- Factors favouring blood transmission :**

- Transfusion: There is a serological window period whatever the screening technique used in blood transfusion centres, and the use of low-sensitivity screening tests would increase the risk of HIV transmission by this route [22].
- Intravenous drug use: the risk of transmission by this route is thought to be increased by the sharing of the syringe and/or needle for injection, the sharing of the preparation (drug), the immediacy of syringe sharing, the partner's injection pattern (more than one injection/day) and finally by the number of intravenous drug users (IDUs) present [17].

**I-1-3-1-3-3- Factors favouring maternal-fk'tale transmission :**

The presence of clinical manifestations of AIDS or a low CD4 count ($<200/mm^3$ ) at the time of pregnancy, a high plasma viral load (high p24 antigenemia, high plasma viremia), recent infection of the mother and intense exposure of the fetus to the body fluids of the infected mother during gestation or delivery are factors that favour transmission of HIV from mother to child [22, 23].

**I-1-3-1-4-The replication cycle :**

The replication stages of the virus are common to all retroviruses. Understanding them is essential in the search for active molecules that block one or more stages in this cycle.

**1st stage:** penetration of the virus into the cell

This stage requires fusion of gp120 across the host cell membrane (this is where fusion inhibitors come into play), followed by recognition by the virus envelope (gp120) of receptors (CD4 molecule) and HIV cell coreceptors (CXCR4 and CCR5). This step is inhibited by CCR5 or CXCR4 inhibitors.

**2nd stage:** reverse transcription of 1'RNA into DNA

The synthesis of proviral DNA results from the copying of viral RNA using reverse transcriptase; during this synthesis, errors are made by this enzyme (1 per 10,000 copies of virus) which are responsible for genetic variability. Reverse transcriptase inhibitors inhibit this step.

**Stage 3:** integration of the viral DNA into the cell genome using viral integrase. This step is inhibited by anti-integrases.

**4th stage:** production of new viral particles with :

- transcription of viral DNA into RNA ;
- then the synthesis of viral proteins from viral messenger RNA
- finally, the assembly of viral proteins after protease activation, a stage inhibited by anti-proteases, and the formation of new viral particles released into the extracellular sector ready to infect other cells.

Virus replication is intense, with around 1 to 10 billion viruses produced every day by an untreated infected person [21].

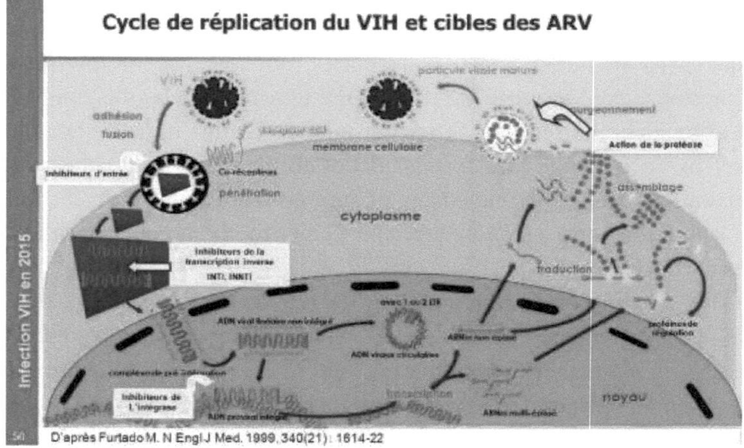


**Figure II: HIV replication cycle with sites of action of ARVs**

### I-1-3-2-Descriptive epidemiology :

**In the world**

Worldwide, 36.7 million [30.8 million - 42.9 million] people were living with HIV; 1.8 million [1.6 million - 2.1 million] people were newly infected with HIV and 1.0 million [830,000 - 1.2 million] people had died of AIDS-related illnesses by the end of 2016 [25].

**In Africa:** according to WHO estimates, 70% of people infected with HIV live in sub-Saharan Africa [13].

**In Mali**

According to Mali's Demographic and Health Survey (EDSM IV), the prevalence of

HIV infection is 1.3% in men and women aged 15 to 49 [26].

**I-1-4-Pathophysiology :**

From the moment of primary infection, the virus actively replicates and spreads throughout the body. Viral reservoirs are thus formed, with the virus integrating into cells (lymph nodes, lymphoid tissue in the digestive tract), enabling it to escape recognition by the immune system.

The virus' target cells are :

- CD4 lymphocytes,
- monocytes/macrophages,
- cerebral microglia cells.

HIV progressively destroys the immune system by infecting CD4 lymphocytes (direct mechanism) and triggering immune activation that leads to multiple pathological immune phenomena, including the destruction of CD4 lymphocytes (indirect mechanism). When CD4 counts fall below 200/$mm^3$ , opportunistic infections occur, with the onset of clinical AIDS.

Because of the early establishment of viral reservoirs and the persistence of minimal replication of the virus, leading to the selection of viruses that evade the host's immune response, even highly effective antiretroviral treatments have not yet been able to eradicate the virus.

In addition, persistent replication of the virus results in constant activation of the immune system, which is insufficient to control HIV and is harmful to many organs (heart, bone, blood vessels, kidneys, etc.).

CD4 cells are rapidly renewed until damage to the central lymphoid organs (thymus) prevents them from regenerating [21].

**I-1-5-Clinical aspects**

**I-1-5-1-The natural history of HIV infection :**

Natural history refers to the natural, predictable order in which the clinical and biological manifestations of HIV infection occur. This is modified by the increasingly early initiation of effective antiretroviral treatment. The spontaneous clinical course of HIV infection is divided into three phases [17].

**I-1-5-1-1-Primary HIV infection :**

The first symptoms appear 10 to 15 days after infection in around 20% of people. They include mononucleosis syndrome, fever, pharyngitis, cervical adenopathy, more rarely aseptic meningoencephalitis, acute myelitis, peripheral neuropathy, facial paralysis, macular exanthema and digestive disorders [20].

These symptoms may be absent, go unnoticed, especially in tropical environments, or be confused with influenza or mononucleosis [27].

All these symptoms improve in about ten days and the patient enters the asymptomatic phase, which lasts 4 to 10 years for HIV-1 and 20 to 25 years for

HIV-2 [27].

Three to 6 weeks after infection with HIV, antibodies become detectable in the serum of infected individuals.

**I-1-5-1-2-The asymptomatic phase :**

This is a clinically latent but biologically active phase. Viral replication is constant, with progressive deterioration of the immune system. This will determine the appearance of the clinical manifestations of the symptomatic phase.

The CD4 count gradually falls over a few years from 500 to 350 per $mm^3$ . This is followed by a phase known as progression, in which the fall in CD4 accelerates to below 200 per mm within a few months[3] . This is a prognostic factor for progression to AIDS, where the viral load is maximal [17].

**I-1-5-1-3-The AIDS phase :**

During this phase, so-called opportunistic infections occur, the main ones being tuberculosis, pneumocystis, toxoplasmosis, cryptococcosis, coccidiosis and candidiasis [27].

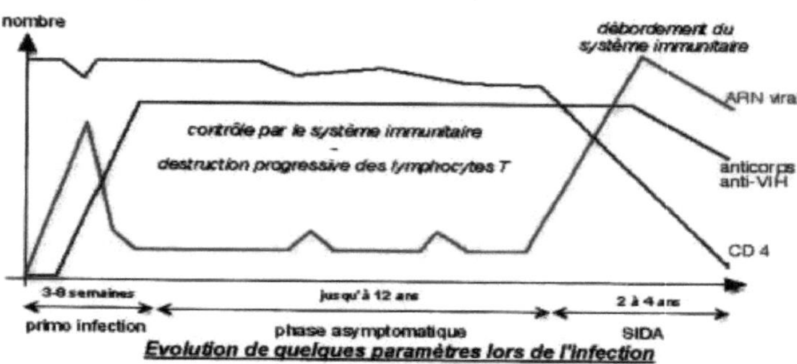


**Figure III: Changes in some parameters during infection** [13, 28].

**I-1-5-2-Clinical manifestations**

**I-1-5-2-1-Dermatological manifestations :**

Dermatological manifestations are observed in almost 80% of AIDS patients and 60% of patients at an early stage.

Oral candidiasis, seborrheic dermatitis, cutaneous dryness, Kaposi's disease, dermatophytosis and mucocutaneous herpes are the most common dermatoses. A particular feature of AIDS in tropical environments is the high frequency of prurigo. Some of these dermatoses have prognostic value, reflecting the extent of the immune deficiency.

The natural history of the dermatological manifestations of AIDS has been profoundly altered by the introduction of effective treatments. The introduction of these treatments can sometimes be accompanied by the appearance of certain dermatoses (herpes zoster, folliculitis), but most of them usually improve spontaneously. Unfortunately, the use of these treatments is also associated with the occurrence of new undesirable effects: drug hypersensitivity syndrome, lipodysmorphic syndrome [2933].

**I-1-5-2-2-Digestive symptoms :**

The digestive tract is one of the main target organs during HIV infection. It is the organ richest in immunocompetent cells in the body and therefore one of the main reservoirs of HIV.

Chronic diarrhoea is the major digestive sign and the second major symptom of AIDS in tropical areas. It may be intermittent, liquid or bloody.

Its etiology is usually infectious, requiring additional tests to identify the causative agent, which is most often *Salmonella*, *Shigella*, atypical mycobacteria, *Cryptospridium*, *Giardia*, *Candida* and *CMV*.

Nausea and vomiting may accompany the diarrhoea. Oral-pharyngeal candidiasis is common and is considered an opportunistic infection in children over the age of one. It is often accompanied by resophagitis.

Since the use of antiretroviral strategies enabling powerful control of HIV replication and restoration of immune function, the frequency of digestive tract infections has fallen dramatically and is now a minor cause of digestive tract disorders [30, 34].

**I-1-5-2-3-Respiratory symptoms**

Frequent and severe, respiratory disease has always played an important role in the spontaneous course of HIV disease, occurring in more than 80% of AIDS patients, but it is also common in latent or overt form at earlier stages.

Clinically, pulmonary signs in AIDS are not very specific. The presentation of pneumopathy is highly variable: insidious and progressively worsening, or very sudden with the onset of respiratory distress within a few hours.

The picture is dominated mainly by a productive cough, often an acute pneumonia with severe hypoxia requiring intensive care. Elsewhere, the clinical picture remains poor in the absence of condensation.

Minor signs may precede certain infections: isolated tachycardia, dyspnoea, chest pain, febricula.

Certain pulmonary complications may be found, such as mycobacteriosis, Kaposi's disease, lymphoma and above all lymphoid interstitial pneumonia, which mainly affects HIV-infected children. Lymphoid interstitial pneumonia is characterised by a cough associated with digital hippocrit, salivary gland hypertrophy and lymphadenopathy.

In the absence of superinfection, fever is absent, and dyspnea and other physical pulmonary signs appear during revolution.

In patients receiving antiretroviral treatment, the incidence of these respiratory pathologies is decreasing in some cases, remaining more or less stable in others; above all, new respiratory manifestations linked to immune reconstitution have appeared and continue to be described [13, 35].

**I-1-5-2-4-Neurological manifestations**

They are not uncommon. In adults in tropical areas, the main symptom is cephalea, which is present in virtually all patients with a neurological syndrome. It is persistent and violent, sometimes accompanied by agitation and insomnia. It is a sign of cerebral cryptococcosis or cerebral toxoplasmosis.

Neurological manifestations are present in 50% of infected children and can be seen even in the absence of any other signs. A distinction is made between :

- encephalopathy with a progressive course marked by psychomotor regression leading to dementia and death;
- encephalopathy evolving in stages, with a good prognosis;
- cerebral growth deficit with microcephaly and cerebral atrophy on CT scan;
- motor disorders with pyramidal syndrome: stiffness is constant, arch reflexes persist after four months and patella clonus is present.
- delayed psychomotor development ;
- ataxia and convulsions.

CSF studies may show anti-HIV antibodies or viral antigens. The disease may progress to spastic quadriplegia with signs of pseudobulbar palsy.

Recent therapeutic advances enabling better control of the infection have modified the frequency of complications in patients being monitored and treated, and in some cases the prognosis of certain opportunistic manifestations has been considerably improved as a result of immune restoration. The nervous system could also act as a reservoir for HIV infection [36-38].

**I-1-5-2-5-Stomatological symptoms:**

They may be indicative of HIV infection. They are dominated by oral mycoses, of which there are several forms:

- The pseudomembranous form is the usual form known as "thrush", which begins with a sensation of cooking or a metallic taste, followed by the appearance of red macules representing diffuse erythematous stomatitis. The gums are usually respected.
- The erythematous form is essentially marked by glossitis.
- Perleche or angular cheilitis is a mucocutaneous localization of the labial commissure.
- The hyperplastic form, which is the pseudo-tumoral aspect of the mycosis.

In addition to oral mycoses, ulcerations of the buccal mucosa, known as chevelous leukoplakia, may be observed [13, 39].

The advent of highly effective antiretroviral therapy, in particular protease inhibitors and non-nucleotide inhibitors, has profoundly altered the landscape of HIV infection [13].

**I-1-5-2-6-Nutritional aspects of HIV infection :**

Undernutrition is and remains one of the major complications of AIDS. Weight loss during HIV infection is marked by its early onset and the rapidity and severity of its progression.

During the course of AIDS, weight loss frequently exceeds
20% of pre-illness weight.

The importance of malnutrition in AIDS led the Center for Diseases Control (CDC) in Atlanta in 1987 to consider a particular syndrome, the wasting syndrome (WS), as an indicator of AIDS. This is characterised by involuntary weight loss of more than 10% of baseline weight, associated with diarrhoea or asthenia and fever in the absence of any infectious or tumour-related etiology. This malnutrition is characterised by a predominant loss of lean body mass, in contrast to pure malnutrition due to protein and energy deficiency [13, 40].

**I-1-5-2-7-Hematological manifestations :**

Hematological abnormalities of all blood lines are common at all stages of HIV infection. During the period of primary infection, hyperlymphocytosis accompanied by mononucleosis syndrome and thrombocytopenia may be transiently observed.

The most frequent haematological abnormalities are cytopenias, which are almost constant at an advanced stage of infection.

They may be due to a complication of the disease or to HIV, in which case they may be central and linked to insufficient medullary or peripheral production. Immunological thrombocytopenia is the most frequent manifestation of the latter type of cytopenia, particularly in patients not yet at the stage of AIDS [13, 41].

**I-1-5-2-8-Nephrological manifestations in HIV :**

The nephrological aspects of HIV disease concern both the renal damage associated with HIV infection and the renal damage caused by the nephrotoxicity of the drugs used in HIV infection.

The nephrological manifestations of the HIV-seropositive patient can be classified into five categories: acute renal failure; electrolyte disorders (dysnatremia, syndrome of inappropriate secretion of ADH, dyskalemia, hypocalcemia or hypercalcemia, hypomagnesemia, hypophosphatemia or hyperphosphatemia); glomerulonephritis associated with HIV infection; nephrotoxicity of antivirals and chronic renal failure [42-45].

**I-1-5-2-9-Other events :**

They are many and varied:

- chronic parotid hypertrophy ;
- cardiomyopathy with left ventricular hypertrophy, especially in children;
- *CMV* chorioretinitis;
- otitis and mastoiditis ;
- thrombocytopenic purpura and autoimmune hemolytic anemia.

It should be noted that HIV has a variable tropism that can affect all organs, resulting in a variety of symptoms [13].

**I-1-5-3-Clinical stages of HIV infection and revised WHO classification of adults and adolescents:**

This is a clinical classification that applies to any seropositive person aged 15 and over [46,47].

**Primary HIV infection**

- Asymptomatic
- Acute retroviral syndrome or symptomatic primary infection

**Stage 1**

- Asymptomatic
- Persistent generalized lymphadenopathy

**Stage 2**

- Moderate unexplained weight loss (< 10% of presumed or measured weight)
- Recurrent respiratory infections (airway infections, sinusitis, bronchitis, otitis media, pharyngitis)
- Zona
- Perleche
- Recurrent oral ulcers
- Prurigo
- Seborrheic dermatitis
- Fungal infections of the nails (onychomycosis)

**Stage 3**

Conditions for which the presumptive diagnosis can be made on the basis of clinical signs or simple tests

- Severe weight loss (> 10% of presumed or measured body weight)
- Chronic unexplained diarrhoea lasting more than 1 month
- Prolonged unexplained fever (intermittent or constant) lasting more than 1 month
- Oral candidiasis
- Hairy tongue leukoplakia
- Pulmonary tuberculosis diagnosed in the previous two years
- Severe bacterial infections (e.g. pneumonia, pyomyositis, joint or bone infection, meningitis, etc.)

❖ Acute ulcero-necrotizing stomatitis/gingivitis/periodontitis

**Conditions for which the diagnosis must be confirmed**

❖ Unexplained anaemia (<8 g/dl) and/or neutropenia (<500/mm3) and/or thrombocytopenia (<50 000/mm3) for more than one month.

**Stage 4**

**Conditions for which a presumptive diagnosis can be made on the basis of clinical signs or simple tests**

❖ Cachectic syndrome

❖ *Pneumocystis jirovecii* pneumonia

❖ Severe recurrent bacterial or radiological pneumonia

❖ Chronic herpes (oro-labial, genital, ano-rectal lasting more than one month)

❖ Resophageal candidiasis

❖ Extra pulmonary tuberculosis

❖ Kaposi's disease

❖ Cerebral toxoplasmosis

❖ HIV encephalopathy

**Conditions for which the diagnosis must be confirmed**

❖ Extra pulmonary cryptococcosis including meningitis

❖ Disseminated infection with non-tuberculous mycobacteria

❖ Candidiasis of the trachea, bronchi or lungs

❖ Cryptosporidiosis

❖ Isosporosis

❖ Visceral herpetic infection

❖ *Cytomegalovirus* infection (retinitis or other than liver, spleen or lymph nodes)

❖ Progressive multifocal leukoencephalopathy

❖ Disseminated mycosis (e.g. histoplasmosis, coccidioidomycosis), penicillosis,...)

❖ Septicemia recurrente a *Salmonella* non typhica

❖ Lymphoma (cerebral or non-Hodgkin's B-cell)

❖ Invasive cervical cancer

❖ Visceral leishmaniasis

**I-1-6-Biological diagnosis**

**I-1-6-1-Serological diagnosis**

**I-1-6-1-1-Screening tests :**

Enzyme-linked immunosorbent assay (ELISA)

❖ Detection of HIV antibodies is based on enzyme-linked immunosorbent assays (ELISA).

❖ The fourth-generation tests used are highly sensitive. They enable the

combined detection of HIV-1 p24 protein and anti-HIV-1 and anti-HIV-2 IgM and IgG antibodies. These tests make it possible to reduce by a few days the window of opportunity during which serology is negative in the course of primary infection.
In addition, so-called rapid tests, which give a response in a few minutes or hours, are also available and can easily be carried out without the need for sophisticated equipment. They are used in emergency situations or exposure accidents.

I-1-6-1-2- **Confirmatory test:** Western-Blot

Western blotting is used to detect antibodies directed against the various HIV proteins: envelope glycoproteins (gp160, gp120, gp41), core proteins encoded by the gag gene (p55, p24, p17) and enzymes encoded by the pol gene (p66, p51, p31).

The criteria for a positive test are those defined by the WHO and consist of the presence of antibodies visually marked by bands against at least two envelope glycoproteins, gp41, gp120 or gp160.

In practice, the serum to be tested undergoes two screening tests of the following type

ELISA (or an ELISA test and a rapid test) detecting antibodies to HIV-1 and HIV-2.

❖ If the result is doubly negative, we can confirm the absence of HIV seroconversion and therefore, except in the case of a strong suspicion of very recent primary infection, the absence of infection by the virus.

❖ If the result is dissociated or double positive, Western blotting is used. The presence of bands on the Western blot that do not meet the criteria for positivity defines an indeterminate Western blot, which may indicate ongoing HIV-1 seroconversion or HIV-2 infection [13, 21].

Western blot is the usual reference method. However, RIPA (Radio Immuno Precipitation Assay) is more sensitive and more specific than Western blot [17].

❖ **The particular situation of recent primary infection**

After infection, HIV multiplies silently in the body for around ten days. This is followed by viremia, which may be accompanied by clinical manifestations of primary infection, preceding seroconversion, i.e. the appearance of antibodies.

In this latent serological phase, PCR, viral isolation and antigenemia detect the primary viremia, making it possible to anticipate the serological diagnosis of infection by a few days. Viral RNA is detectable 8 to 10 days after infection, p24 antigenemia around 15 days after infection and serum antibodies 22 to 26 days after infection. Seroconversions occurring more than 3 months after exposure are exceptional (<1%) [17].

**I-1-6-2-Virus quantification :**

**Determination of viral load**

Plasma viral RNA (plasma viral load), a sign of viral replication, can be quantified by genomic amplification (PCR). The detection threshold for this technique is currently between 20 and 200 copies/ml, depending on the technique. Viral load is of vital importance in monitoring HIV infection:

❖ It is a prognostic factor for the progression of untreated HIV infection: the higher the viral load, the faster the decline in CD4 lymphocytes and the greater the risk of disease progression;

❖ it is an essential part of monitoring antiretroviral treatment.

The aim of antiretroviral treatment is to achieve and maintain an undetectable viral load. An isolated rise in viral load, if it remains below 1000 copies/ml, may be observed without pathological significance. Any value above the repeated fagon threshold should prompt an investigation into the cause of this virological failure [17].

**I-1-7-Management of HIV/AIDS infection in Mali**

**I-1-7-1-Psychosocial care**

There is no way of predicting an individual's reaction to being diagnosed as HIV seropositive. Shock is a normal reaction to life-threatening news and can take many forms (anger, anxiety, fear, guilt, denial, suicide). The psychosocial approach to treatment involves providing information, psychological, social and emotional support, allowing feelings to be expressed and discussed, and encouraging the establishment of social and medical care [46,48].

**I-1-7-2-Specific treatment:** based on antiretroviral drugs (ARVs).

**I-1-7-2-1-Nucleoside reverse transcriptase inhibitors (NRTIs)**

They were the first ARVs to be marketed and are natural nucleoside derivatives. They are the cornerstone of combination therapy. Table 1 lists the nucleoside inhibitors [46, 47].

**Tableau I: The list of nucleoside inhibitors available in Mali with their dosage and most frequent toxicity** [46, 47].

| Designation | Dosage | Most frequent toxicity | Comments |
|---|---|---|---|
| Abacavir (ABC)<br>Cp 300 mg Box / 60 | • Adult: 300 mg /12 h<br>• In case of liver failure :<br>• Light: 300 mg/12h<br>• Moderee : to be avoided<br>• Severe: contra-indicated<br>• 600 mg x 1/24h is also approved. | - Hypersensitivity reactions | - After screening for the HLA-B*5701 allele (in Caucasians) and only if negative (unless no other therapeutic alternative is available for the patient).<br>- consultation every 15 days for the first 2 months of treatment ;<br>- warning card given to the patient ;<br>- definitive stop if allergic |

| | | | reaction or if such a reaction cannot be eliminated;<br>- and return of all remaining product;<br>- if reintroduced: hospital consultation. |
|---|---|---|---|
| Lamivudine (3TC) 150 mg tablet<br>Box / 60<br>Suspension 10 mg/1ml<br>Bottle/240ml<br>300 mg tablet<br>Box /30 | > 50 mL/min => 300 mg/24h<br>26 to 49 mL/min => 150 mg/24h<br>"25 mL/min } => once 150 mg hemodialysis } then 25 to 50 mg/24 h | - Generally well tolerated. | |
| Tenofovir (TDF) Tablet 300 mg Bte/30 | With a meal, depending on creatinine clearance :<br>> 50 mL/min => 1 cp /24 h<br>30-49 mL/min => 1 cp /48 h<br>10-29 mL/min => 1 cp /72-96 h<br>on dialysis => 1 tablet after 12 hours of dialysis | - Proximal tubulopathy (including Fanconi syndrome). | Exceptionally (if difficult to swallow), the tablet may be diluted in at least 100 mL of water, orange juice or grape juice. |
| Zidovudine (AZT)<br>Tablet 300 mg, Box / 60<br>solution 100mg/10ml<br>Bottle/200ml 200 mg/20ml Inj Bte/5amp | according to creatinine clearance (in mL/min) : -> 26: 300 mg/12 h - < 26 and hemodialysis: 150 mg/12 h | -Severe anaemia or neutropenia - Severe gastrointestinal intolerance - Lactic acidosis | |

**I-1-7-2-2-Non-nucleoside reverse transcriptase inhibitors (NNRTs)**

They are potent and selective, but inactive against group O HIV-2 and HIV-1.

**Tableau II: List of non-nucleoside reverse transcriptase inhibitors transcriptase available in Mali with dosage and toxicity the most frequent** [46, 47].

| Designation | Dosage | Most frequent toxicity | Comments |
|---|---|---|---|
| Efavirenz (EFV)<br>Gel 200, Box / 90; tablet 600 mg Box /30<br>Susp 30mg/ml<br>Bottle/180ml | 600 mg/24h in a single daily dose | Persistent and severe central nervous system toxicity | at bedtime, with or without food |
| Nevirapine (NVP)<br>Tablet 200 mg<br>Oral solution 50mg/5ml<br>Bottle/240ml | - For the first 14 days: 200mg a day.<br>- Then: 200 mg/12 h, unless a rash occurred during the first | -Hepatitis<br>-Hypersensitivity reaction<br>Severe or life-threatening rash (Stevens-Johnson and Lyell syndrome) | |

| | period.<br>- If > 7 days: reintroduce according to the same schedule. | | |
|---|---|---|---|

**I-1-7-2-3-Protease inhibitors (P.I.) :**

**Tableau III: The list of protease inhibitors available in Mali with the most frequent dosage and toxicity** [46,47].

| **Designation** | **Dosage** | **Most frequent toxicity** | **Comments** |
|---|---|---|---|
| Ritonavir RTV<br>- Softgel capsule 100 mg, Box / 84 | In association with other PIs :<br>• 100 mg /24h with atazanavir (300 mg /24h)<br>• 100 mg /12h with darunavir (600 mg /12h), | Digestive disorders: nausea, vomiting, diarrhoea, abdominal pain, dyspepsia, anorexia | |
| Atazanavir (ATV) tablet 300 mg Box/ 30 | 300 mg/24h | | In combination with other antiretroviral agents - In HIV-1-infected adults - Taking into account resistance tests and previous treatment. |
| Lopinavir (LPV)/Ritonavir (r) Comp: 200mg/50mg 100mg/25 mg Suspension 80/20 mg/ml Bottle/60ml (400mg+100mg)/5ml Bottle/60ml | 2 tablets at 200/50 mg/12h, with or without a meal - or (5 mL of oral solution)/12h | | do not chew, cut or crush the tablets. |
| Raltegravir RAL Tablet 400mg<br>B/120 | 400mg/12h | | |

| Darunavir DRV Tablet 400mg B/120 | 2pills/12h | | |
|---|---|---|---|

### I-1-7-2-4-Adult ARV combinations available in Mali

**Tableau IV: List of ARV combinations in Mali (adults)**

| N° | Designation | Dosage |
|---|---|---|
| 01 | 3TC+AZT+ABC<br>(150 + 300 + 300) mg tablet, Box/60 | 1 tablet/12h |
| 02 | TDF+3TC+EFV<br>(300 + 300+ 600) mg tablet Box/60 | 1 tablet/24h in the evening |
| 03 | AZT+3TC<br>(300 + 150) mg, Box / 60 | 1 tablet/12h |
| 04 | AZT/3TC/NVP | 1 tablet/12h |
| 05 | LPV/r | See above |

### I-1-7-3-The objective of ARV treatment

The aim of antiretroviral treatment is to achieve and maintain an undetectable viral load (cv) in order to restore immunity, thereby increasing life expectancy and improving patients' quality of life [46].

### I-1-7-4-Principles of ARV treatment in Mali

It is a lifelong treatment, requiring excellent compliance from patients and intensive monitoring by healthcare staff. Antiretroviral treatment is a triple therapy generally combining two inhibitors

nucleoside/nucleotide reverse transcriptase inhibitor (NRTI) to a non-nucleoside reverse transcriptase inhibitor (NNRTI) or a protease inhibitor.

Fixed combination therapies should be favoured to encourage compliance and reduce the cost of treatment for the country.

The molecules used must appear on Mali's list of essential medicines or benefit from special authorisation and will necessarily be prequalified by the WHO and a qualification.

### I-1-7-4 Indications for ARV treatment in adults and adolescents

Antiretroviral treatment is indicated as soon as HIV+ status is discovered [46].

### I-1-7-5-Therapeutic regimens

A first-line regimen is considered to be any first-line regimen prescribed for a patient who has not received any antiretroviral treatment. Any substitution in the event of intolerance, for example, is also considered a first-line regimen.

A second-line regimen is any regimen prescribed after first-line treatment has failed.

**I-1-7-5-1-First-line regimens for HIV-1**

They combine two NRTIs and one NNRTI of preferred fagon.

The preferred first-line treatment is as follows:

**Tenofovir (TDF) + Lamivudine (3TC) + Efavirenz (EFV) 400**

NB: treatment with the EFV 600 will continue until the EFV 400 is acquired.

The following alternative plans are possible:

**Zidovudine (ZDV, AZT) + Lamivudine (3TC) + Nevirapine (NVP)**
**Zidovudine (ZDV, AZT) + Lamivudine (3TC) + Efavirenz (EFV)**
**Tenofovir (TDF) + Lamivudine (3TC) + Nevirapine (NVP)**

**I-1-7-5-2-Special cases**

**a. Treatment of HIV/Tuberculosis co-infection**

Antiretroviral treatment should be given as a matter of course to anyone living with HIV and presenting with active tuberculosis, regardless of their CD4 T lymphocyte count.

There are drug interactions between NNRTIs or PIs and rifampicin. Nevirapine (NVP) is not recommended due to its additive hepatotoxicity with anti-tuberculosis drugs. Efavirenz (EFV) 600 is the preferred NNRTI.

The proposed 1st line diagrams are :

1^ere^ option: **Tenofovir (TDF) + Lamivudine (3TC) + Efavirenz (EFV)600**

2^eme^ option: **Zidovudine (AZT) + Lamivudine (3TC) + Efavirenz (EFV)600**

**b. Management of patients infected with HIV-2 or co-infection HIV-1 and HIV-2 (or group O HIV-1 infected patients)**

The choice of treatment excludes non-nucleoside reverse transcriptase inhibitors, which are not effective against HIV-2 or group O HIV-1.

Treatment regimens combining nucleoside/nucleotide reverse transcriptase inhibitors with a boosted protease inhibitor (PI/r) or 3 NRTIs will be used.

The preferred first-line treatment is as follows:

**Tenofovir (TDF) + Lamivudine (3TC) + Lopinavir / Ritonavir (LPV/r)**

The therapeutic alternatives in the event of toxicity, intolerance or drug interaction are as follows:

**Zidovudine (AZT) + Lamivudine (3TC) + ATV/r or**
**Zidovudine (AZT) + Lamivudine (3TC) + Abacavir (ABC)**
**Tenofovir (TDF) + Lamivudine (3TC) + ATV/r**

**I-1-7-5-3-Second-line treatment**

The 2nd line regimen must include at least 2 new molecules, one of which must be from a different family to those used in the first line. Lamivudine (3TC) must always be maintained in 2nd line.

In the event of confirmed HIV 1 and 2 treatment failure in the first line, the following preferred second-line regimen is recommended:

2 nucleoside/nucleotide inhibitors + 1 boosted protease inhibitor

The preferred PIs are : Lopinavir/ritonavir (LPV/r), Atazanavir/ritonavir (ATV/r)

**I-1-7-5-4-Third-line treatment**

Patients in 2nd-line virological failure should be managed according to the results of the resistance genotyping test.

DRV/r + DTG (or RAL) ± 1-2 NRTIs

DRV/r + 2 NRTIs ± NNRTI

**I-1-7-5-5-Therapeutic regimen for pregnant women**

The regimen to be proposed for pregnant women will be prophylactic therapy according to one of the following regimens:

| **AZT or TDF + 3TC + NVP**<br>**AZT + (3TC or FTC) + EFV**<br>**(AZT or TDF) + 3TC + (LPV/r or IDV/r or SQV/r or ATV/r)** |
|---|

**I-1-7-5-Monitoring adult and adolescent patients**

**I-1-7-5-1-Patient information and preparation**

Given the chronic nature of ARV treatment and the importance of compliance for its effectiveness, each patient will receive therapeutic education and psychological and social support as required before starting treatment. During subsequent consultations, therapeutic education and psychological and social support will be provided on a regular basis.

Intra-family screening should be offered as a matter of course, so that the status of the whole family is known.

Secondary prevention should be discussed with the patient's sexual partners.

**I-1-7-5-2-The initial assessment and follow-up of the patient**

**I-1-7-5-2-1-Pre-therapeutic assessment**

It is clinical and para-clinical.

A thorough clinical examination includes weight, height, BMI, blood pressure, tuberculosis assessment and pregnancy screening in women of childbearing age.

Depending on the patient's clinical condition and the technical platform, a minimum assessment will be requested before treatment is initiated:

- Blood count (CBC)
- Transaminases (ALAT)
- Glycemia
- Proteinuria (quantitative or qualitative)
- Creatinemia and calculation of clearance,
- Front chest X-ray

- Search for BAARs in cases of suspected TB and/or GenExpert
- HBs antigen; total anti-HbC antibodies (IgG + IgM)
- Anti-HCV or HCV antibodies
- Rhesus grouping
- Viral load
- TCD4 lymphocyte count.
- Patient education is essential.

**I-1-7-5-2-2-The follow-up report :**

**Day 15**: assessment of compliance and tolerance, transaminases in patients on Nevirapine, proteinuria and creatinemia in patients on Tenofovir (depending on technical facilities).

**Month 1:** clinical examination (including weight, assessment of tuberculosis), assessment of compliance and the following biological work-up (depending on the technical platform):

- Blood count (CBC)
- Transaminases (ALAT)
- Proteinuria
- Creatinemie/Clairance
- Glycemia
- Systematic search for BAARs

After the 1st month of treatment, clinical monitoring will continue on a monthly basis until the 3eme month mark.

**NB:** in patients on TDF, regular monitoring of creatinemia and clearance every month until 3eme months, then quarterly.

**Month 2:** clinical examination (including weight, BP measurement, tuberculosis assessment) and assessment of compliance and tolerance.

**Month 3:** clinical examination (including weight, BP measurement, assessment of tuberculosis), assessment of compliance, and the following biological work-up (depending on the technical platform):

- Blood count (CBC)
- Transaminases (ALAT)
- Proteinuria
- Creatinemia/clearance
- Glycemia.
- Cholesterol and triglycerides
- Testing for BAARs in the presence or absence of signs of tuberculosis

**Month 6, Month 12 and every 6 months**: clinical examination (including weight, BMI assessment, BP measurement, tuberculosis assessment), assessment of compliance and tolerance, clinical efficacy, tuberculosis assessment, biological work-up which may include :

- ❖ Blood count (CBC)
- ❖ Transaminases (ALAT)
- ❖ Glycemia
- ❖ Proteinuria (quantitative or qualitative)
- ❖ Creatinemia and calculation of clearance,
- ❖ Front chest X-ray
- ❖ Testing for BAARs in cases of suspected tuberculosis
- ❖ HBs antigen, total HbC antibodies (IgG + IgM)
- ❖ Anti-HCV or HCV antibodies
- ❖ Viral load
- ❖ TCD4 lymphocyte count.

Evaluation of the immunovirological response (CD4 T lymphocyte count and CV) during ARV treatment should be carried out every six months or at least once a year and as required [46].

**I-2-Physiology and hydrolytic metabolism**

The equilibrium of the internal environment, or homeostasis, is essential for the proper functioning of multicellular organisms. The evolution of living beings, and in particular the transition from the aquatic to the terrestrial environment, was only made possible by species adapting to meet the constraints imposed by changes in their environment. The gradual disappearance of the surrounding liquid environment led primitive organisms to surround themselves with an aqueous microenvironment in order to survive outside the water.

In humans, the cell compartment, bounded by the plasma membrane, is bathed in extracellular fluid, a dilute solution whose osmolality and pH are tightly regulated, and a relatively minor deviation from these parameters can cause serious dysfunction.

Hydrolytic disorders are common to all medical and surgical pathology. Their diagnosis and treatment can avert serious, sometimes life-threatening, complications. This is an area where analysis and understanding of physiology are fundamental [49].

In addition to their endocrine function, the kidneys are also responsible for purifying the body's waste products and regulating the internal environment. This second function concerns water and most of the electrolytes, the quantity or concentration of which must be regulated at a stable level to avoid sometimes major clinical problems.

The tubules are responsible for regulation. Regulation of the quantity or concentration of water and electrolytes in the internal environment results in a remarkably stable electrolyte concentration in the plasma.

In physiology as in physics, the regulation of a variable involves a control loop between a parameter measured in a direction such that this variation tends to bring the parameter measured closer to the normal value.
The kidney uses numerous control loops to regulate the internal environment. As a result, an electrolyte disorder occurs whenever the regulation of the water or electrolyte concerned no longer functions normally, either because the functioning of the control loop is impaired or because its regulatory capacity is exceeded [49].
Hydrolytic disorders, when they appear in PLWHA of any origin, can complicate the patient's clinical condition. Hyponatremia is most common in PHAs [50].

**I-2-1-Water distribution in the internal environment :**

Schematically, water represents 60% of body weight: 40% in the intracellular sector (ICS) and 20% in the extracellular sector (ECS), which itself includes the interstitial (15%) and vascular (5%) sectors. Water content is lower in women and decreases with age [49, 51].
Other sub-compartments could also be distinguished, such as lymph, CSF, serosites, etc., but we prefer to include them in the "interstitial" medium for greater ease of understanding [49].

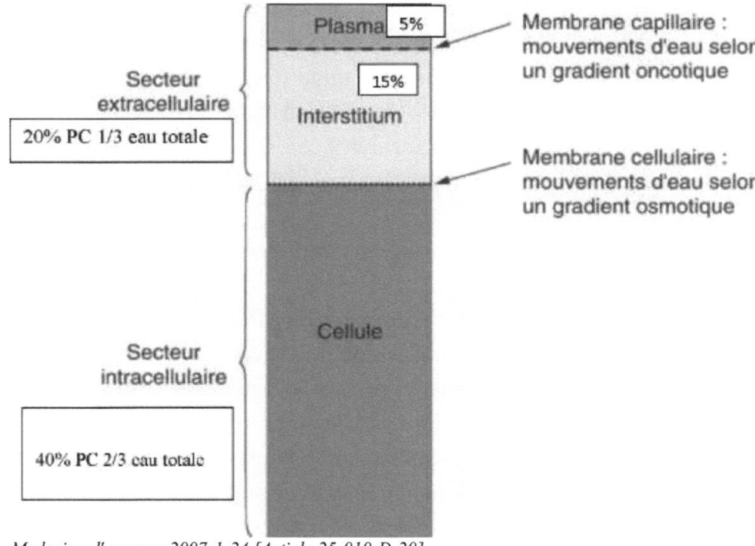


*EMC - Medecine d'urgence 2007:1-24 [Article 25-010-D-20]*

**Figure IV:** Diagram showing the different compartments of the organism.

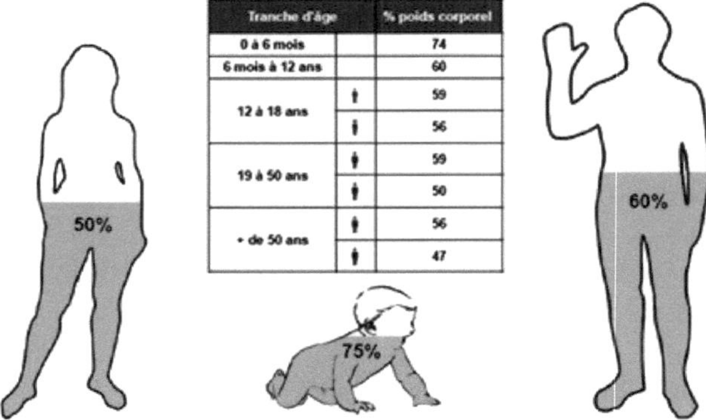


| Tranche d'âge | | % poids corporel |
|---|---|---|
| 0 à 6 mois | | 74 |
| 6 mois à 12 ans | | 60 |
| 12 à 18 ans | | 59 |
| | | 56 |
| 19 à 50 ans | | 59 |
| | | 50 |
| + de 50 ans | | 56 |
| | | 47 |

*EMC - Medecine d'urgence 2007:1-24 [Article 25-010-D-20].*

**Figure V: Variation in body water content according to sex, age and body fat**

### I-2-2-The composition and distribution of electrolytes in the body's various compartments

#### I-2-2-1 Composition of the internal environment :

Solutes are divided into electrolytes and non-electrolytes. Non-electrolytes generally have covalent bonds that prevent them from dissociating and therefore do not carry an electric charge. Most non-electrolytes are organic molecules: glucose, lipids, creatinine, urea. Electrolytes, on the other hand, are chemical compounds that dissociate into ions. As ions are charged particles, they can conduct electricity, hence their name.

Electrolytes include inorganic salts, organic and inorganic acids and bases, and certain proteins [52].

#### I-2-2-2-Ion distribution in the different compartments :

The extracellular compartment is subdivided into several sub-compartments.

The intravascular sector corresponds to plasma and represents 30 to 35 ml/kg of body weight, i.e. 25% of extracellular fluid. Water represents 93% of the plasma volume in the vessels and heart chambers. The substances dissolved in plasma water are ionised (cations and anions) and non-ionised (urea, glucose). The main plasma cation is sodium ($Na^+$). This is the determinant of plasma osmotic pressure. Plasma also contains macromolecules (albumin 40 g/l).

The interstitial sector comprises the space surrounding the cells. The water mass represents 15% of the body mass, or 150 ml/kg of weight. Its composition is almost identical to that of plasma.

The intracellular sector accounts for 40% of body water and potassium (K+) is the dominant cation [52].

**I-2-3-Movement of fluid between the body's different compartments**

**I-2-3-1-Definitions :**

Osmosis is the principle of diffusion of a solvent between two compartments of different concentration through a membrane. The solvent moves from the less concentrated medium to the more concentrated one.

Plasma osmolarity is the number of osmoles of a solution per litre expressed in milli-osmoles per litre.

Calculated plasma osmolarity (OsmPc) is equal to the sum of all plasma osmotic substances (active or inactive) measured on the blood ionogram. **OsmPc= 2xNa + glycemia + urea=280-295mosm/l**

Plasma osmolality is the concentration in milli-osmoles per kilogram of water in the plasma compartment. It eliminates the volume variations associated with proteins and lipids. Its normal value is between 280 and 295 mosm/kg of water [51].

Plasma tonicity is the force that determines the net movement of water across the membrane. It corresponds to the sum of the osmotically active substances in a solution. Any variation in tonicity in one compartment results in a variation in volume in the compartment concerned. Plasma tonicity is the sum of all osmotically active ions [52].

**Plasma tonic=2xNa + glycemia =275-290 mosm/l**

Although all molecules and solutes contribute to the osmotic activity of the liquid, the osmotic power of electrolytes is greater than that of non-ionising molecules. Water therefore moves or diffuses in the direction of the osmotic gradient, i.e. from the compartment with the lowest osmolalinity (low ion concentration) towards the compartment with the highest osmolalinity (higher ion concentration). Plasma osmolality is equal to 290 mosmol/l [52].

**I-2-3-2-Gibbs and Donann equilibrium :**

Due to the existence of non-diffusible ions in a compartment alongside diffusible ions, there is a transmembrane osmotic pressure gradient. This is known as colloido-oncotic pressure or oncotic pressure.

In human physiology, Donann's law is found in blood capillaries, where proteins are non-diffusible anions responsible for an oncotic pressure that retains water in the capillaries.

In addition, Gibbs and Donann's law renders the distribution of ions between cells and interstitium unequal, thus ensuring a transmembrane potential difference [52].

**I-2-3-3-The body's water sectors :**

The movement of water between the plasma and the interstitial medium is governed by 2 forces:

- hydrostatic pressure. It tends to force the water out of the plasma into the interstitial medium.
- an oncotic pressure (proportional to the protein content) which causes water to enter the plasma from the interstitial medium.

The flow of water between the intracellular medium and the extracellular medium is regulated by osmotic pressure. Water moves to balance the intracellular and extracellular osmolalites. Water moves from the medium with the lowest osmolality to the medium with the highest osmolality (less concentrated to more concentrated) [51].

**I-3-Electrolyte measurement :** This is based on the ionogram.

**I-3-1-Definition :**

The ionogram is a medical biology laboratory test which analyses the concentration of electrolytes in a body fluid (blood, urine, cerebrospinal fluid). These electrolytes are salts, acids and bases capable of dissociating in solution to form ions.

The blood or plasma ionogram is the measurement of the main plasma electrolytes cations (sodium, potassium, calcium, magnesium) and anions (chlorine, bicarbonate or alkaline reserve, phosphate, proteins). It is often performed in conjunction with renal function parameters (urea, creatinine) [53].

**I-3-2-Types of blood ionogram:** there are several types.

- Simple ionogram: sodium ($Na^+$); potassium ($K^+$); chlorine ($Cl^-$).
- Complete ionogram: simple + bicarbonate ($HCO_3^-$) and proteins.
- Extended ionogram: complete + calcium ($Ca^{++}$) and phosphates.

**I-3-3-The method :**

Blood is taken on an empty stomach, venous or arterial blood (if gasometry) in a dry tube (serum) or with an anticoagulant (lithium heparin for plasma). Avoid using a tourniquet that is too tight or pumping your hands during sampling (haemolysis). The sample should be taken to the laboratory quickly to avoid haemolysis [54].

The main technique is potentiometry using an ion-selective electrode specific to the dose electrolyte (measurement of the potential difference created by the solution containing the reference ions) [53].

**I-3-4-Results and standards :**

- Sodium= 135-145 mmol/l
- Potassium= 3.5-5 mmol/l
- Chlorine= 95-105 mmol/l

- Bicarbonates=22-30 mmol/l
- Calcium=2.25-2.5 mmol/l
- Magnesium=0.75-1 mmol/l
- Phosphates=0.8-1.35 mmol/l
- Total protein= 65-75 g/l [54].

**I-4-Anomalies in the simple blood ionogram :**

These are essentially dysnatremia and dyskaliemia.

**I-4-1-Dysnatremia :**

**I-4-1-1-Sodium regulation:** The Na ion is one of the most important balances for maintaining homeostasis. In all its forms, it represents more than 90% of extracellular ions. As it does not readily cross plasma membranes, it is actively transported by Na/K pumps [49].

There are three main regulatory mechanisms:

- Aldosterone is the main factor regulating extracellular sodium, although in its absence 80% of Na+ is still reabsorbed in the kidney. Aldosterone causes active Na reabsorption in the distal convoluted tubules and collecting ducts. Aldosterone is produced by the glomerular zone of the corticosurrenal gland. Its production is activated mainly via the juxta glomerular apparatus by the renin angiotensin system. This is triggered by a drop in arterial pressure or filtrate osmolarity, and vice versa.
- Baroreceptors in the aortic arch and neck vessels "monitor" the maintenance of blood flow by measuring blood pressure. In the event of a fall in blood flow, impulses are sent to the kidney via the hypothalamus and the sympathetic nervous system, which reduces its glomerular filtration rate, reabsorbing water and Na.
- Finally, hypothalamic osmoreceptors detect variations in solute osmolarity and communicate the information to the hypothalamus.

In response to these influxes, the neurohypophysis adapts its secretion of antidiuretic hormone: an increase in Na triggers the release of ADH, allowing it to be diluted and vice versa [49].

Sodium is an accessory intracellular cation with a concentration of only 10 to 15 mmol/l of cellular water.

Sodium is maintained in the extracellular sector by an active mechanism, with the concentration gradient and the negative electric field tending to cause sodium to diffuse into the cell. Sodium is permanently expelled from the cell by a membrane-based mechanism, the "sodium pump", which pumps out an amount of sodium equal to that which the electrochemical gradient causes to diffuse in.

This active rejection of sodium is linked to the maintenance of potassium in the cell and depends on metabolic activity, the functioning of which is impaired by cold, anoxia and other specific metabolic inhibitors.

The sodium balance is controlled by dietary intake and excretion via the various elimination routes. The mass of exchangeable sodium undergoes constant renewal. Inputs are exclusively digestive. Intestinal absorption is rapid, around three minutes, and virtually complete.

This passive absorption is very important in quantitative terms, as it involves dietary sodium and sodium from digestive, intestinal and especially colonic secretions.

Digestive elimination is negligible (10 mmol/day) and sweat losses are very low (1 to 2 mmol).

The main route of elimination is via the urine. Sodium balance is essentially controlled by the kidney. Various regulatory factors are involved, including mineralocorticoids [49].

Natremia generally provides information about the hydration status of the intra-cellular sector.

- Hypernatremia corresponds to an increase in extracellular osmolarity, which leads to a withdrawal of water from the intracellular sector and therefore intracellular dehydration.
- Hyponatremia most often corresponds to a decrease in extracellular osmolarity, which leads to a leakage of water into the intracellular sector and therefore intracellular hyperhydration.

As the cells most sensitive to variations in their hydration are neurons, the clinical symptoms of cell hydration disorders are above all neurological, and treatment must be progressive, as correction that is too abrupt can be very serious.

**I-4-1-2-Hyponatremia :**

It is defined as a natremia of less than 135 mmol/l.

Hyponatremia means intra-cellular hyperhydration.

The onset of hyponatremia may be acute or chronic. The absolute value is less important than the rate of onset, which must be determined as precisely as possible [52].

**I-4-1-2-1 Classification of hyponatremia :**

Depending on plasma osmolality, a distinction is made between hypertonic hyponatremia, isotonic hyponatremia (pseudohyponatremia) and hypotonic hyponatremia (true hyponatremia) [52, 55].

**I-4-1-2-1-1-Hypertonic hyponatremia or false hyponatremia :**

They are due to the accumulation in plasma of substances other than sodium. These substances are active osmoles (glucose, glycerol, mannitol) inducing hyperosmolarity and hypertonicity. (plasma osmolalite > 295 mosmol/l)

**Corrected natremia = [(Na) observed + (glycemia - 5)] /3**

**I-4-1-2-1-2-Isotonic hyponatremia or pseudohyponatremia :**

They are due to the presence in plasma of abnormally high quantities of non-aqueous substances, as seen in hyperlipidemia and hyperprotidemia. They are iso-osmotic and isotonic. (plasma osmolality = 280-295 mosmol/l)

**I-4-1-2-1-3-Hypotonic hyponatremia or true hyponatremia :**

They are hypotonic (plasma osmolality < 280 mosmol/l) and associated with intracellular hyperhydration. Depending on their mechanism of onset, they are associated with certain changes in extracellular volume (ECV).

**I-4-1-2-1-3-1-Hypotonic hyponatremia with normal VEC [52, 55] :**

These are dilution hyponatremias. They are due to hydric inflation secondary to insufficient loss of water in relation to inputs. The sodium capital is preserved so that intracellular hyperhydration (ICH) is associated with normal blood flow. They are more common in the syndrome of inappropriate ADH secretion (SIADH) found in paraneoplastic syndromes (ectopic tumour secretion of ADH (or ADH-like substance): bronchial carcinomas, prostate and digestive cancers, lymphomas, etc.)..); cerebral lesions (infectious: meningitis, meningo-encephalitis, abscesses; ischemic or haemorrhagic cerebral vascular accidents; multiple sclerosis, polyradiculonevritis, acute porphyria, cranial trauma);
pulmonary pathologies (bacterial and viral pneumopathies; respiratory insufficiency; iigiic' , tuberculosis, cancers, asthma...); mechanical ventilation; the post-operative period (stress, pain, severe nausea syndromes); endocrinopathies (hypothyroidism, cortico-surrenal insufficiency, prolactin adenoma) and the use of drugs (carbamazepine; psychotropic drugs : haloperidol, phenothiazines, IRS-type antidepressants (fluoxetine ++), tricyclic antidepressants, MAOIs, drugs (amphetamines or ecstasy); emetogenic drugs: cyclophosphamide, vincristine, vinblastine..; drugs that potentiate the effect of ADH: hypoglycemic sulphonamides (chlorpropamide), theophylline, clofibrate, exogenous intake of ADH or ADH analogues (oxytocin).

**I-4-1-2-1-3-2-Hypotonic hyponatremia with reduced ECV [52, 55] :**

They are also known as depletion hyponatremia. They are due to water and sodium losses, but the sodium deficit exceeds that of water. In this case, the sodium and water pools are initially reduced, but hypovolemia, which stimulates ADH secretion, combined with an exogenous intake of water, helps to aggravate the hypotonic hyponatremia. There is extracellular dehydration with intracellular hyperhydration (DEC+HIC).

They are common during digestive losses (vomiting, diarrhoea, fistula, occlusion) or skin losses (burns) and salt loss syndrome (SLS) in patients with cerebral lesions.

**I-4-1-2-1-3-3-Hypotonic hyponatremia with increased ECV [52, 55].**

These are hyponatremias caused by hydrosodium inflation. They are due to water and salt retention, with water predominating. There is both intra- and extra-cellular hyperhydration (global H). They are more common in congestive heart failure, decompensated cirrhosis, nephrotic syndromes and hypoprotidemia.

**I-4-1-2-2-Clinical manifestations of hyponatremia [52, 55] :**

Symptoms vary depending on how quickly hyponatremia sets in.

In the case of slow, progressive onset, the picture is asymptomatic for a long time. These include :

- a change in general condition ;
- progressive behavioural problems;
- serious neurological disorders in cases of profound hyponatremia.

In the event of a rapid onset of symptoms, exceeding the cells' capacity for adaptation, particularly in the brain, the symptoms are digestive and neurological:

- disgust for water; nausea and vomiting ;
- cephalea; obnubilation, confusional or delusional syndrome, coma, seizures, rarely cerebral involvement.

NB: Neurological signs can be difficult to distinguish from those of the underlying disease.

Neurogenic pulmonary rearrhythmia has been reported during exercise-induced hyponatremia in marathon runners.

**I-4-1-2-3-Treatment of hyponatremia [52, 55] :**

The treatment of hyponatremia includes etiological treatment and symptomatic treatment, which consists of reducing the relative or absolute excess of water.

In all cases, water restriction of 500 cc/d may be recommended.

Symptomatic treatment varies according to the VEC:

- Normal ECV (pure ICH): fluid restriction alone.
- VEC decreases (DEC+HIC): 0.9% Na Cl intake to normalise the extracellular sector
- Increased ECV (global hyperhydration): fluid restriction combined with a loop diuretic (furosemide) to normalise the extracellular sector.

The recommended rate of correction is as follows:

A rate of increase in natremia of 1 mmol/L/h is quite sufficient, without exceeding a total increase of 8 to 12 mmol in the first 24 hours. In any case, an increase in natremia of 2 mmol/L/h over the first 12 hours is not acceptable. Correcting hyponatremia too quickly does not give the cells time to regain the solutes lost, and the result is cellular dehydration responsible for centropontine myelinolysis (discrete tremor, tetraplegia, facial diplegia, loss of lateral gaze) or osmotic demyelinisation. Alcohol- and drug-dependent patients are particularly at risk.

Symptomatic hyponatremia (Na <120 mmol/L, coma or convulsions) indicates that the capacity for cell volume reduction has been exceeded and warrants aggressive management. The following schema can be proposed:

- infusion of hypertonic sodium chloride (1 to 2 g/h, 10% hypertonic NaCl solute), correcting the natremia by no more than 1 to 2 mmol/L/h over the first 3-4 hours until clinical symptoms have resolved, but not exceeding 8 to 12 mmol/L over the first 24 hours. Monitoring in an intensive care unit is essential;
- in the second stage, treatment reverts to that of asymptomatic hyponatremia [52, 55].

**I-4-1-3-Hypernatremia :**

It is defined as a natremia of more than 145 mmol/l. It is responsible for intracellular dehydration. It reflects an inadequate adjustment of the fluid balance.

**I-4-1-3-1 Classification of hypernatremia :**

They are classified into 3 types: hypervolemic hypernatremia, isovolemic hypernatremia and hypovolemic hypernatremia [52].

**I-4-1-3-1-1-Hypervolemic hypernatremia or exceptionally excessive sodium :**

They are most often due to excessive sodium intake from iatrogenic causes (resuscitation errors) or insufficient dilution of milk in children.

The clinical picture combines extracellular hyperhydration and intracellular dehydration (ECH + ICD).

**I-4-1-3-1-2-Isovolemic hypernatremia or water deficit :**

They are due to water loss, predominantly in cases of osmotic polyuria or central or nephrogenic diabetic insipidus: intracellular dehydration (ICD) is pure.

**I-4-1-3-1-3-Hypovolemic hypernatremia or hydrosode deficit:**

They are due to hypotonic losses from the digestive tract, the skin, but more often from the kidneys as a result of osmotic polyuria, diuretics or, in the case of hyperglycaemia, hypercalcemia. Their compensation is insufficient, leading to extra- and intracellular dehydration (DEC + DIC).

**I-4-1-3-2-Manifestations of hypernatremia :**

**a-The symptomatology varies greatly depending on the rapidity of onset and intensity of the deficit, and is usually marked by intra- and extra-cellular dehydration.**

Extracellular dehydration: skin folds, hypotension, flat veins, oliguria.

Intracellular dehydration: intense thirst, fever, dry mucous membranes, muscular fatigue, neurological disorders such as agitation, obnubilation, convulsions and coma, with a risk of subdural hematoma in infants.

**b- Biological signs**

Signs of haemoconcentration: increased haematocrit, protidemia, uremia with functional renal failure. Plasma hyperosmolalite (>290mmol/l).

**I-4-1-3-3-Treatment of hypernatremia :**

Treatment is guided by two principles: firstly, to gradually correct the deficit in water capital, and secondly, to treat the cause of the mechanism initiating water loss. Hypernatremia of 180 mmol/L or more has a poor prognosis.

1. **Correcting the water deficit:** This is based on simple rules.

a. **Assessing the water capital deficit**

Assuming that total water loss is solely responsible for the increase in hypernatremia, the variation in hypernatremia is inversely proportional to the variation in total water. The water capital deficit is calculated using the following formula:

**Water deficit = 0.6x weight (kg) x [(Natremia (mmol/l)** /140) **-1]**

The figure obtained is a useful estimate that must always be placed in its clinical context.

b. **Prescribing food intake for the first 24 hours**

Oral supplements are only given if the patient is fully conscious and the deficit is small.

In the event of impaired alertness, fluids should be administered via the parenteral route: subcutaneous administration is only possible if the daily quantity to be infused is less than or equal to 2 litres; above this quantity, fluids should be administered via the peripheral venous route.

The choice of the type of solution to be infused depends on the clinical condition:

- in the event of hypovolemia: isotonic saline solution,
- in the absence of hypovolemia: semi-isotonic saline with 4.5 g/L Na Cl, or 2.5 or 5% glucose solute without Na Cl.

In cases of symptomatic ждиё hypematremia, natremia may be lowered by 1 mmol/L/hour up to 145 mmol/L. When hypernatremia has been present for a long time, the rate of correction should not exceed 10 mmol/L/d to avoid inducing cerebral redeme and convulsions.

2. **Treatment of the mechanism initiating total water loss**

It is essential and depends on the etiology in question:

- in the case of diabetic insipidus: treatment with desmopressin;

- in the case of diabetic hyperosmolar coma: prescription of insulin according to the usual recommendations [55].

**I-4-2-Dyskalemia**

Potassium is the most abundant univalent cation in the body and the main cellular cation. As such, it is the major determinant of intracellular osmolality.
Potassium is also a cofactor in many metabolic processes. Potassium disorders give rise to numerous complications.
In general, the body is fairly well protected against hyperkalaemia (except in patients with renal failure). It is much more sensitive to potassium losses [56].

**I-4-2-1-Potassium distribution in body tissues :**

Extracellular fluids contain just 2% of potassium (1% in the interstitial sector and 1% in plasma).
Intracellular fluids contain 98% of potassium, 75% of which is found in the muscles. The concentration of potassium there reaches 140 mmol/l of tissue.
Total body potassium is estimated at 55 mmol/kg in men and 49 in women (lower adipose tissue content). For a 70 kg man, total body potassium is estimated at 3500-4000 mmol.
The absolute quantity of potassium, as well as the ratio between its extra- and intracellular concentrations, are the major determinants of the resting membrane potential. In this respect, potassium participates, along with other ions (calcium, magnesium) and pH, in membrane excitability [56].

**I-4-2-2-Clinical consequences of muscle potassium levels**

- Any significant muscle destruction (myolysis) tends to create hyperkalemia.
- Any potassium disorder tends to create functional impairment of both smooth and striated muscles, leading in particular to potentially serious changes in myocardial electrogenesis [56].

**I-4-2-3-Movements of potassium**

Potassium homeostasis involves maintaining :

- of a body potassium pool, i.e. the balance between intake and losses (external balance);
- a concentration gradient between the intracellular space, which is very rich in potassium, and the extracellular space, which is very poor in potassium (internal balance). This gradient is essential for the polarisation of the cell's basal membranes, the basis of cell function. Its strict equilibrium is imperative.

♦ **) External scales :**

- Dietary intake: 50 to 150 mmol/day (2 to 6 g). The main source is fruit and vegetables (raw). Unlike sodium, this intake can never be reduced to zero.
- Elimination: 90% is renal. Fecal losses represent less than 10%; skin loss (1%) is negligible.

♦ ) **The internal balance:** this relates to potassium transfers. Several factors affect intra-extracellular exchange.

♦ Insulin: facilitates the combined entry of glucose and potassium into many cells. It therefore plays a part in regulating kalinity.

Any increase in kaliemia increases insulin secretion, which favours potassium entry into the cell and attenuates the intra/extracellular imbalance.

♦ Activation of the Na-K-ATPase membrane pump: stimulated by insulin.

♦ Catecholamines: Modify potassium transfer.

- alpha agonists reduce cellular uptake and increase kalemia;
- beta agonists increase it; this property is used to treat hyperkalaemia.

♦ Acid-base balance: As with the tubule (of which cells are only a special case), acidosis tends to drive potassium out of the cell [56].

**I-4-2-4-Regulation of potassium in the body and potassium balance:** The intracellular concentration of potassium is 100 to 140 mmol/l, whereas normal kaliemia is 3.5 to 5 mmol/l. The internal potassium balance consists of regulation of potassium between extra- and intracellular media with the aim of maintaining normal kaliemia. The external balance consists of a balance between potassium inputs and outputs.

Inputs come from the diet (75 mmol). They are normally balanced by an equivalent renal excretion [52].

**I-4-2-5-Lhypokalemia :**

It is defined as a fall in plasma potassium concentration below the lower normal limit of 3.5 mmol/l. It can be explained by two main mechanisms which, in certain circumstances, may be combined: transfer and depletion [52,55].

**I-4-2-5-1 Classification of hypokalemia :**

**I-4-2-5-1-1-Transfer hypokalemia :**

It results from excessive extracellular potassium entering cells, mainly liver and muscle cells. The total amount of potassium remains the same but the ratio (Ke/Ki) decreases significantly. The factors likely to cause the transfer are: alteration of the acid-base balance, excess insulin or beta-2 adrenergic agonists, catecholamines, theophylline and WESTPHAL disease (familial periodic paralysis).

**I-4-2-5-1-2-Depletion hypokalemia :**

It results from an imbalance between potassium input and output. The imbalance is in favour of the outflow. It is always accompanied by a decrease in the total quantity of potassium and the Ke/Ki ratio changes downwards. There are two types of leakage: extrarenal or digestive (profuse diarrhoea, vomiting, abuse of laxatives, biliary, pancreatic or intestinal fistulas, etc.) and renal [52].

### I-4-2-5-2-Manifestations of hypokalemia :

Symptoms are the result of abnormalities in membrane polarisation affecting neuromuscular tissues (skeletal and cardiac striated muscle, smooth muscle). They depend on :

- the acute or chronic onset of hypokalemia;
- of its intensity.

The severity of hypokalemia results in particular from cardiac rhythm disorders or respiratory muscle damage.

**a) Neuromuscular signs :**

- Minor signs: muscle fatigue, paresthesia, cramps, myalgia.
- Major signs :
- Tetany attacks;
- Muscular paralysis. These initially affect the lower limbs, then become global (paraplegia, tetraplegia). They are flaccid and accompanied by the abolition of idiomuscular reflexes, while that of osteotendinous reflexes is inconstant. There is no sensory disturbance. They are reversible.

> Complications :

- Paralysis may extend to the trunk, upper limbs and respiratory muscles.
- Exceptionally, extreme hypokalemia can lead to anatomical damage (rhabdomyolysis), rather than just functional damage.

**b) Digestive signs:**

Smooth muscle damage can lead to digestive sluggishness (meteorism, nausea, constipation).

A more serious disorder (paralytic ileus, with functional occlusion) is possible. Its occurrence in a postoperative context (absence of gas crisis) generally indicates a resuscitation error (uncompensated digestive aspiration).

**c) Cardiac signs :**

These are essentially electrocardiographic changes.

These abnormalities partly dictate the course of treatment, and are rapidly reversible under treatment, with a rebound in kalemia, even before the potassium deficit has been fully corrected. They are classified into five stages.

Stage I: normal electrocardiogram

Stage II: lengthening of the PR

Stage III: ST sub-shift

Stage IV: inversion or disappearance of the T wave

Stage V: appearance of the U wave

When kalemia is below 2.5 mmol/l, electrocardiographic changes degenerate into ventricular rhythm disorders (ventricular extrasystoles, ventricular tachycardia, ventricular fibrillation). Hypokalemia increases the toxic effect of digitalis.

**d) Kidney signs:** kaliopenic nephropathy.

Prolonged and massive potassium deficiency can lead to tubular damage, characterised by a disturbance in potassium concentration. Kalemia is usually <2 mmol/l. There is a polyuric-polydipsic syndrome that is unresponsive to the administration of ADH.

Histological study shows vacuolation of proximal and sometimes distal tubular cells. Renal failure of varying severity may occur.

**I-4-2-5-3-Clinical forms**

**a) Acute hypokalemia :**

The rapidity of potassium loss leads to a more rapid reduction in the extracellular pool (and kalinity) than intracellular loss. The ratio of intracellular to extracellular K is increased. The result is an increase in resting membrane potential and membrane hyperpolarisation, leading to neuromuscular hypoexcitability. Symptoms are therefore essentially muscular, skeletal or cardiac. The main danger is rhythm disorders. Other factors (calcium, pH) are also involved.

**b) Chronic hypokalemia :**

As potassium loss is slower, it occurs proportionately between the two compartments. A transfer of intracellular potassium attenuates the fall in kaliemia. Functional changes in the basal membranes are reduced.

With equal kalinity, potassium loss is much better tolerated than when it is acutev Muscular signs are moderate (asthenia, cramps) or absent. However, kaliopenic nephropathy is more likely to develop [56].

**I-4-2-5-4-Treatment of hypokalemia :**

**a) Goals**

Treat the cause, increase intakes or reduce kaliuresis as appropriate.

**b) Resources**

Depending on the case, potassium is supplied via the diet, potassium tablets or intravenous infusions.

Potassium-sparing diuretics are used to reduce kaliuresis.

**c) Indications**

In cases of severe hypokalaemia (<2.5 mmol/l): kalaemia must be raised to 3 mmol/l. Intake is at a rate of 10 to 20 mmol/h of K+ (< 1g/h) without IV bolus.

In moderate cases (>2.5 mmol/l with normal ECG), potassium supplementation is authorised by :

- Food: bananas, oranges, grapefruit, milk, potatoes, spinach, tomatoes, meat, etc.
- potassium chloride tablets (Kaleorid, Diffu-K, Kalienor)

In cases of hyperkalemia, treatment is based on potassium-sparing drugs (spironolactone, triamterene, amiloride, etc).

**d) Results and monitoring**

Depending on whether the hypokalemia is acute or chronic, the therapeutic efficacy is monitored by ionograms and/or electrocardiograms repeated at variable intervals.

Preventive measures are instituted to avoid recidivism [52, 55, 56].

**I-4-2-6-Hyperkalemia :**

It is defined as an increase in plasma potassium concentration above 5 mmol/l. Hyperkalemia can be explained by two mechanisms: a defect in elimination and a transfer phenomenon [55].

Hyperkalaemia rarely occurs in normal subjects, as the body's defences prevent the consequences of excessive potassium levels:

- by increasing cellular uptake (role of insulin and catecholamines);
- by the increase in renal excretion. In the case of acute overload, the increase in excretion begins as early as the 6th hour. In the case of chronic overload, increased excretion can counterbalance a food intake of 500 mmol per day.

Hyperkalaemia can therefore only occur in the following cases:

- massive and brutal cellular lesion (tissue lysis) resulting in massive passage of potassium into the extracellular compartment (the kidneys have no time to intervene);
- renal failure, particularly acute renal failure^;
- combination of these two conditions [56].

**I-4-2-6-1-Classification of hyperkalaemia: I-4-2-6-1-1-Hyperkalaemia due to impaired renal elimination:**

The reduction in the kidney's capacity to eliminate potassium may result from an acute or chronic reduction in glomerular filtration, primary or secondary hypoaldosteronism, or selective impairment of the renal tubules' capacity to extract potassium.

**I-4-2-6-1-2-Transfer hyperkalemia :**

It may occur in the event of massive elimination of intracellular potassium or suppression of the essential mechanism of tolerance to an acute potassium load represented by cellular entry. It may be found in acute acidosis, cellular lysis and drug intake [52].

**I-4-2-6-2-Clinical manifestations of hyperkalemia :**

From cardiac rhythm disorders, the most frequent clinical situations are renal insufficiency and rhabdomyolysis. The latter is manifested by the following symptoms: myalgia, muscle weakness, pain on pressing the muscles; muscle contractures, cramps or even paralysis; urine coloured reddish-brown [52].

**I-4-2-6-3-Treatment of hyperkalemia :**

Treatment must be started as soon as possible. This is a therapeutic emergency, so for a rapid effect in redistributing potassium:

Glucose combined with insulin: 100 ml of 30% serum glucose in a bolus and 10 IU insulin; this results in a 0.6 mEq/l reduction in kalemia in 15 minutes. The maximum effect is reached in 30-60 minutes. After the bolus, the use of a continuous infusion is discussed.

02 agonists (salbutamol) combined with insulin-glucose maximise the effect. It is administered as a continuous infusion of 0.5 mg over 15 minutes. It reduces kalemia by 1mEq/l after 1 hour. The mechanism of resistance to this treatment is unknown.

Loop diuretics (furosemide) or ion exchange resins (Kayexalate*) per os (30-60g) or enema (100-200g). The onset of action is 2 hours, with a maximum effect of 6 hours. There is a risk of colonic necrosis in 1.8% of cases.

Dialysis: this is the method of choice. It results in a 2 mEq/l decrease in kalemia over the first 3 hours [52].

**I-5-Electrolyte disorders in HIV-infected patients**

Hyponatremia is the most common electrolyte disorder in HIV-infected patients and may result from a variety of physiological disorders [50, 57]. Excessive digestive or cutaneous sodium loss, sodium leakage from tubulointerstitial renal disease, syndrome of inappropriate antidiuretic hormone (ADH) secretion due to opportunistic infections, renal insufficiency and administration of hypotonic solutions are among the causes of hyponatremia in these patients. Hypernatremia is less common, and may also be due to dehydration. Foscarnet-induced diabetic insipidus has been described [50, 58].

Hypokalemia may be due to incoercible vomiting and diarrhoea or due to potassium leakage following treatment with amphotericin B [50, 59]. In contrast, hyperkalemia usually results from hyporenemic hypo-aldosteronism or adrenal insufficiency [50, 60]. Elevated kalimia is also observed in more than 75% of patients receiving high doses of sulfamethoxazole-trimethoprim [50, 61].

Foscarnet, DDI and pentamidine can cause hypocalcemia or hypomagnesemia, often associated with hypocalcemia. Other causes of hypomagnesemia in HIV-infected patients are magnesium loss due to treatment with amphotericin B. Hypercalcemia may occasionally occur following granulomatous diseases or lymphomas [50].

Hypouricemia is observed in more than 22% of patients with AIDS and results from the high fractional excretion of uric acid in HIV-infected patients, for reasons that are unclear [50].

## 2 MATERIALS AND METHODS

### II-1- Equipment

#### II-1-1. Setting and location of the study :

Our study took place in the Infectious Diseases Department of the Centre Hospitalier et Universitaire (CHU) du Point "G" (Bamako, Mali).

This department is one of the country's key sites for the management of AIDS cases. The department has a capacity of 30 beds and receives an average of 32 patients per month. HIV patients account for 80-90% of hospital admissions.

#### II-1-2. The study population :

Our study focused on HIV patients admitted to the infectious diseases department at Point "G".

**a. Sampling :**

We carried out an exhaustive sampling by including all HIV patients who met our inclusion criteria and who had been hospitalised during the study period. The size of the sample was not fixed at the outset.

**b. Inclusion criteria**

We included in the study patients who had performed at least one simple blood ionogram and who met the following criteria:

- age over 18 ;
- hospitalized in the Infectious Diseases Department and having an available and usable medical file;
- positive HIV serology ;
- on ARVs or not.

**c. Non-inclusion criteria**

Patients whose :

- HIV serology was indeterminate or negative;
- the medical file was not available or could not be used;
- No blood ionogram was performed.

**d. Definitions [54] :**

Simple blood ionogram: natremia, kaliemia and chloremia.

Normal natremia: 135-145 mmol/l

Hyponatremia: natremia < 135 mmol/l

Hypernatremia: natremia > 145 mmol/l

Normal kalemia: 3.5-5 mmol/l

Hypokalemia: Kaliemia <3.5 mmol/l

Hyperkalemia: Kaliemia >5 mmol/l

### II-2-Methods

#### II-2-1-Type of study :

This was a retrospective, cross-sectional, descriptive and analytical study covering a six-year period from 1 January 2011 to 31 December 2016.

**II-2-2-Procedure of the study :**

Patients were included on the basis of hospital medical records. The search for patients with at least one simple blood ionogram was carried out in the archives of the Infectious Diseases Department. A request was made to the major of this department for access to the archived hospital medical records.

**II-3-Data collection :**

**II-3-1-Data collection method**

The data were collected using a survey form which we filled in after analysing the patients' medical records.

**II-3-2-Data collected**

For each patient included, we looked for the following parameters:

**a - socio-demographic data:** age, sex, ethnicity, marital status, residence, professional activities.

**b- antecedents**: medical, surgical, eating habits, other associated treatments.

**c-clinical data:** reason(s) for hospitalisation, gastrointestinal disorders (diarrhoea, vomiting); vitals: temperature, pulse, respiratory rate, blood pressure and body mass index (BMI); signs of dehydration; neurological signs: irritability, depression, consciousness disorders (Glasgow score), seizures, intracranial hypertension; smooth muscle signs: constipation, ileus; striated muscle signs: fatigue with muscle hypotonia.

**d-biological data :**

- biological tests based on the determination of the main ionic constituents of the blood;
- haematological tests based on the haemogram
- biochemical tests based on creatinine, protein, blood glucose, albumin and triglyceride levels.
- viro-immunological data based on HIV type, absolute value of CD4 T lymphocytes, viral load if possible.

**e-electrocardiographic data:** looking for cardiac rhythm and repolarisation disorders.

**f-therapeutic data :**

- antiretroviral treatment;
- duration of treatment ;
- tolerance of treatment ;
- Other medicines taken before or during treatment, including: sulphamethoxazole-trimethoprim, fluconazole, amphotericin B, aciclovir, rifampicin, isoniazid, ethambutol, pyrazinamide, digitalis, diuretics and insulin.

**g-revolution data :**

- length of hospital stay ;
- the outcome of hospitalisation in terms of discharges, deaths and discharges without medical advice.

The clinical, biological, electrocardiographic, therapeutic and evolution data were those available on admission and during hospitalisation.

**II-3-3-Techniques for carrying out certain examinations :**

**a-HIV serology**

HIV serology was carried out using Determine rapid tests (the first of their kind in Europe).

intention) and ImmunoComb II HIV 1 & 2 ($2^{eme}$ intention).

**b-Count of CD4+ T lymphocytes**

CD4+ T cell counts were performed using a FACSCount flow cytometer.

**c-Ion dosing:** an automatic electrolyte analyser with an ion selective electrode (ISE) model 5 was used.

**d- Assessment of nutritional status:** nutritional status has been assessed using the body mass index (BMI). According to the WHO, the results of this measurement are :

> Normal BMI = [18.5; 24.9];

> Severe ждиё malnutrition: BMI< 16 ;

> Moderate ждиё malnutrition: BMI = [16, 18.4] ;

> Over-nutrition: BMI= [25; 40].

**II-4-Statistical data entry and analysis :**

The data were entered and analysed using IBM SPSS Statistics Version 21 software.

The statistical tests used were parametric tests (mean, standard deviation) and non-parametric tests (Chi-2 test (/2), and Fisher's exact test for tables with theoretical numbers < 5), with a significance threshold for $p < 0.05$.

Word processing was carried out using Microsoft Word 2010 and Microsoft Excel 2010.

**II-5-Ethical considerations :**

The files were analysed in strict compliance with confidentiality. In fact, the identity of each patient was kept anonymous, as the individual survey form did not include the patient's name and surname, but an anonymous number, which was used to enter the data. The files were then returned and filed in the archives immediately after processing.

This data will be used solely for the purpose of improving patient management and preventing complications associated with electrolyte disorders. The results obtained will be communicated to the health authorities and published if necessary.

**II-6-The GANTT chart :**

| Periods<br>Activities | 02/01/2017 to 31/01/2017 | 01/02/2017 to 05/06/2017 | 06/06/2017 to 05/09/2017 | 06/09/2017 to 16/10/2017 | 17/10/2017 to 29/11/2017 |
|---|---|---|---|---|---|
| Bibliographic research | ■ | | | | |
| Drawing up and correcting the protocol | | ■ | | | |
| Data collection and analysis | visit | | ■ | | |
| Redaction of memory | | | | ■ | |
| Correction of document | | | | | ■ |
| Submission | | | | | |

## 3 RESULTS

**III-1-Descriptive study :**

**III-l-l-General data :**

During our study period, 2286 patients were admitted to the infectious diseases department, 90% of whom had HIV/AIDS. We included 126 out of 2058 PLWH treated or not on any ARV treatment. The flow chart and figure VI below show the general data.

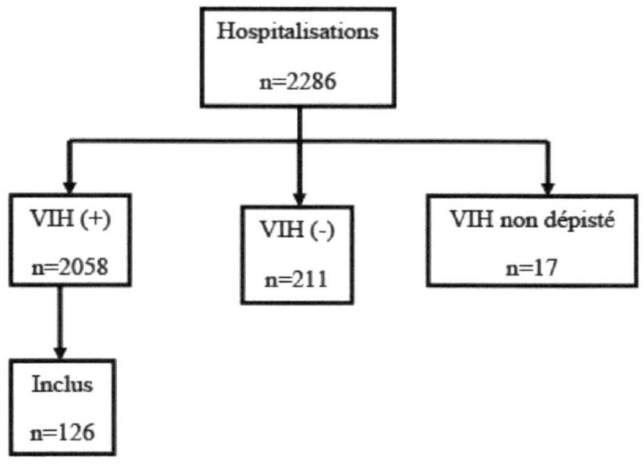


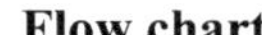

**Flow chart**

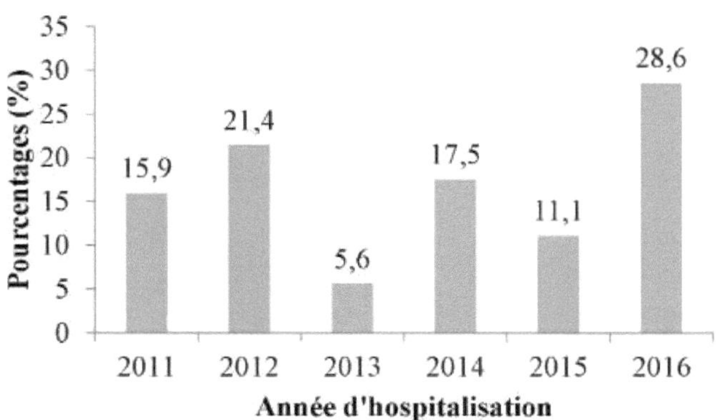


**Figure VI: Distribution of patients by year of hospitalisation**

Patients included in 2016 predominated with 28.6%, followed by those included in 2012 (21.4%).

**III-1-2-Sociodemographic data :**

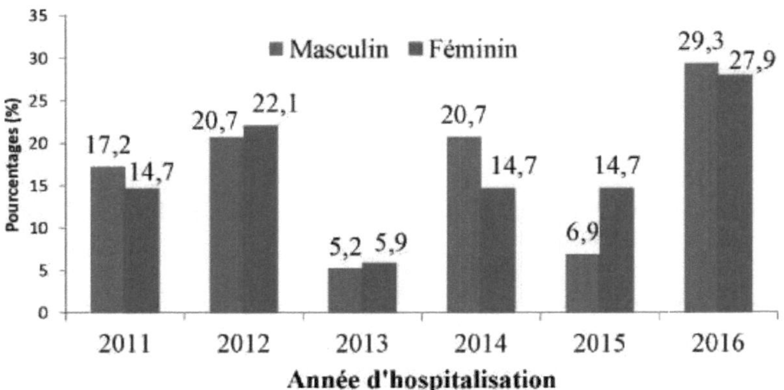


**Figure VII: Breakdown of patients by sex and year of hospitalisation**

In 2016, the number of patients included was higher for both sexes, with 29.3% for men compared with 27.9% for women.

**Table V: Socio-demographic characteristics of the study population**

| Features | Number (n=126) | Percentage (%) |
|---|---|---|
| **Age** | | |
| 18-27 years old | 11 | 8,7 |
| 28-37 years old | 34 | 27,0 |
| 38-47 years old | 32 | 25,4 |
| Age 48-57 | 31 | 24,6 |
| 58 and over | 18 | 14,3 |
| **Gender** | | |
| Male | 58 | 46,0 |
| Female | 68 | 54,0 |
| **Residence** | | |
| District of Bamako | 86 | 68,2 |
| Inland (Regions) | 35 | 27,8 |
| Outside the country | 5 | 4,0 |
| **Marital status** | | |
| Single | 13 | 10,3 |
| Marie | 91 | 72,2 |
| Widower | 15 | 11,9 |
| Divorce | 7 | 5,6 |
| **Profession** | | |
| Commergant | 27 | 21,4 |
| Menagere | 43 | 34,1 |
| Civil servant | 11 | 8,7 |

| | | |
|---|---|---|
| Uniform wearer | 6 | 4,7 |
| Cultivator | 10 | 7,9 |
| Artisan | 17 | 13,5 |
| Driver | 12 | 9,5 |

Our study population was predominantly female (54%). The mean age of the patients was 43 ±12 years, with extremes ranging from 22 to 70 years. Patients living in Bamako were the most numerous (68.3%). Married patients represented 72.2% of the study population. The most common occupation was housewife (33.3%).

**IH-1-3-Clinical data:a**

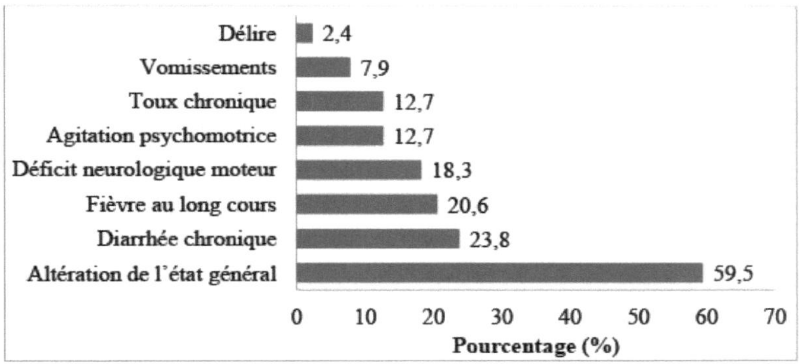


**Figure VIII: Breakdown of patients by reason for hospitalisation**

The main reason for hospitalisation was deterioration in general condition (59.5%), followed by chronic diarrhoea (23.8%) and long-term fever (20.6%).

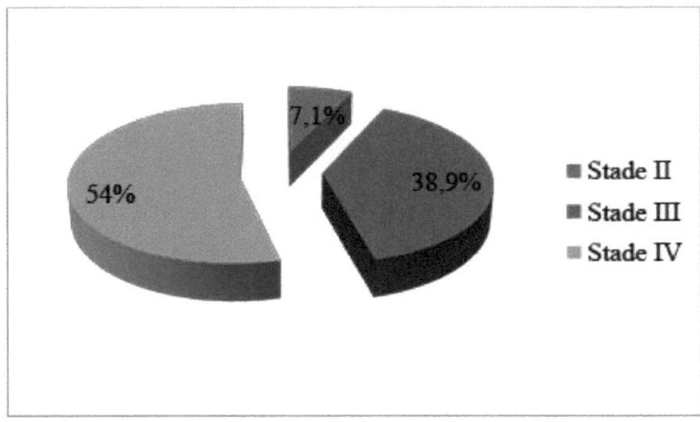


**Figure IX: Distribution of patients according to WHO clinical stage of AIDS**

Stage IV patients were the most numerous (54%).

**Table VI: Distribution of patients according to clinical signs**

| Clinical signs | Workforce | Percentage (%) |
|---|---|---|
| **Constant anomalies** | | |
| Polypnee | 96 | 76,2 |
| Fever | 58 | 46 |
| Arterial hypotension | 55 | 43,7 |
| Tachycardia | 28 | 22,2 |
| Hypothermia | 22 | 17,5 |
| State of shock | 8 | 6,3 |
| HTA | 5 | 4,0 |
| **Digestive signs** | | |
| Anorexia | 75 | 59,5 |
| Diarrhoea | 54 | 42,9 |
| Vomiting | 37 | 29,4 |
| Constipation | 2 | 1,6 |
| **Neurological signs** | | |
| Consciousness disorders | 44 | 34,9 |
| Motor neurological deficit | 26 | 20,6 |
| Convulsive seizures | 11 | 8,7 |
| Trembling | 10 | 7,9 |
| Delire | 8 | 6,3 |
| Depressive syndrome | 1 | 0,8 |
| **Signs of intracranial hypertension** | | |
| Cephalees rebelles | 18 | 14,3 |
| Uncontrollable vomiting | 7 | 5,6 |
| **Muscular signs striae** | | |
| Fatigability | 21 | 16,7 |
| Muscle hypotonia | 7 | 5,6 |

The clinical signs in order of frequency were polypnoea (76%), anorexia (59.5%), fever (46%), arterial hypotension (43.7%), diarrhoea (42.9%), disturbed consciousness (34.9%) and vomiting (29.4%).

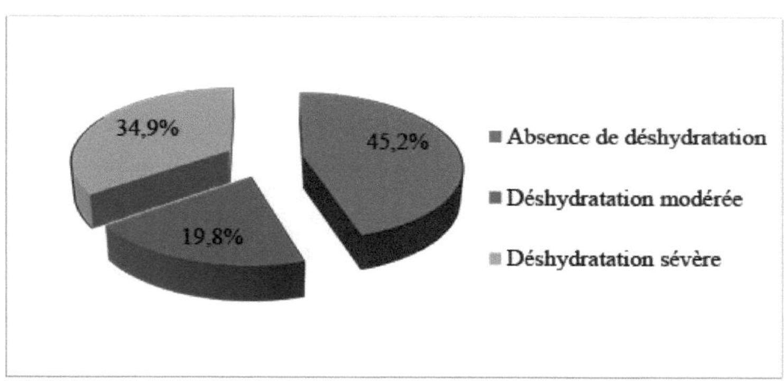


No dehydration
Moderate dehydration
Severe dehydration

**Figure X: Distribution of patients according to hydration status**

Patients were dehydrated in 54.8% of cases, including 34.9% of severe cases.

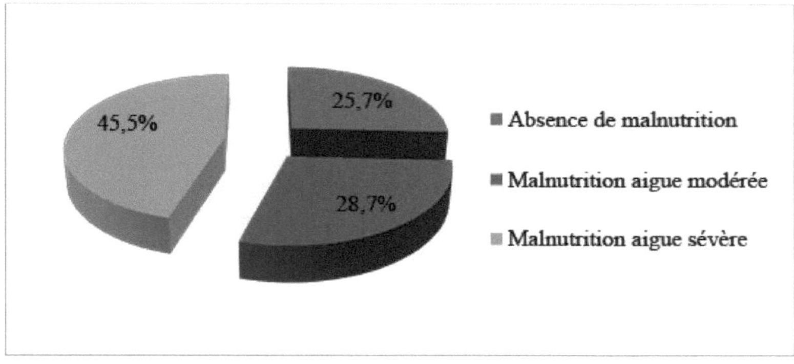


Absence of malnutrition
Moderate acute malnutrition
Severe acute malnutrition

**Figure XI: Distribution of patients according to nutritional status**

Patients were malnourished in 74.2% of cases, including 45.5% of severe cases.

**Table VII: Breakdown of patients by pathology diagnosed**

| Diagnosed diseases | Workforce | Percentage (%) |
|---|---|---|
| **Oral candidiasis** | **69** | **54,8** |
| **Cerebral toxoplasmosis** | **33** | **26,2** |
| **Tuberculosis** | **25** | **19,8** |
| Malaria | 23 | 18,2 |
| Lower urinary tract infections | 20 | 15,9 |
| Non-tuberculous bacterial pneumonia | 19 | 15,1 |

| | | |
|---|---|---|
| Bacterial and/or parasitic diarrhoea | 17 | 13,5 |
| Isosporosis | 3 | 2,4 |

The most frequently diagnosed pathologies were oral candidiasis (54.8%), followed by cerebral toxoplasmosis (26.2%) and all forms of tuberculosis (19.8%).

**IH-1-4-Biological and electrocardiographic data :**

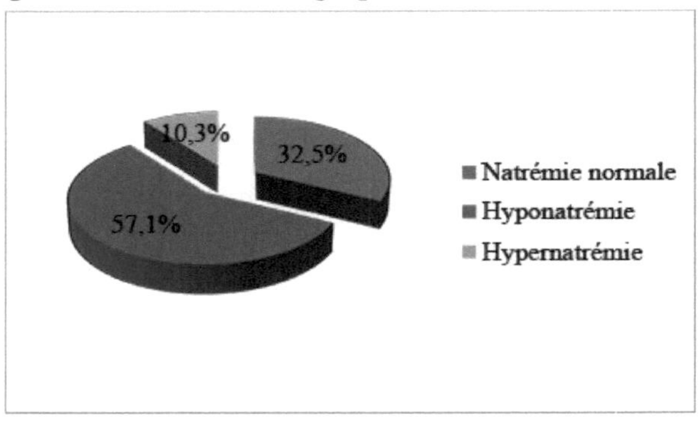


- Normalatremia
- Hyponatremia
- Hyperatremia

**Figure XII: Distribution of patients according to natremia**

Patients had dysnatremia in 67.4% of cases (57.1% hyponatremia and 10.3% hypernatremia). The mean natremia was 133.06±12.16 mmol/l, with extremes of 83.00 and 166.00 mmol/l.

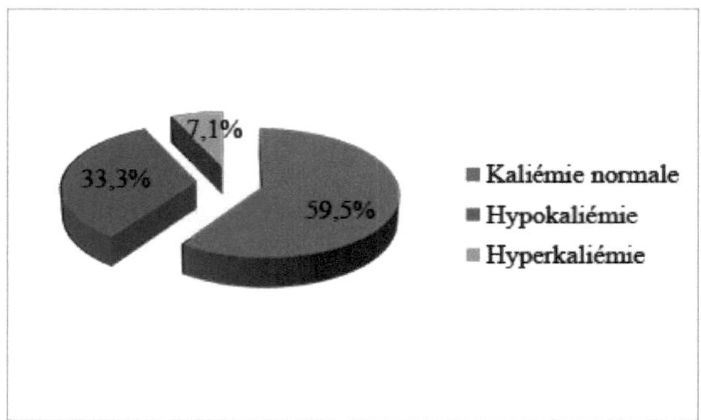


- Normal kaliemy
- Hypokalemia
- Hyperkalemia

**Figure XIII: Distribution of patients according to kalemia**

Patients had dyskalaemia in 40.4% of cases (33.3% hypokalaemia and 7.1% hyperkalaemia). The mean kaliemia was 3.89±1.15 mmol/l with extremes ranging from 1.60 to 9.00 mmol/l.

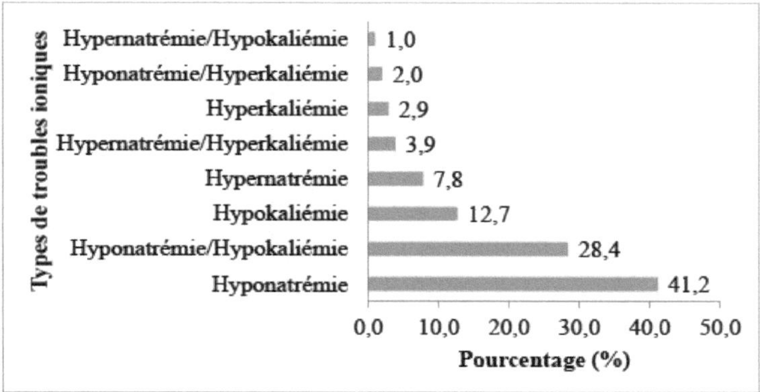


**Figure XIV: Frequency of electrolyte disorders**

Hyponatremia predominated in 41.2% of cases, of which 50% were depletion hyponatremia and 50% dilution hyponatremia. There were no cases of inflation hyponatremia.

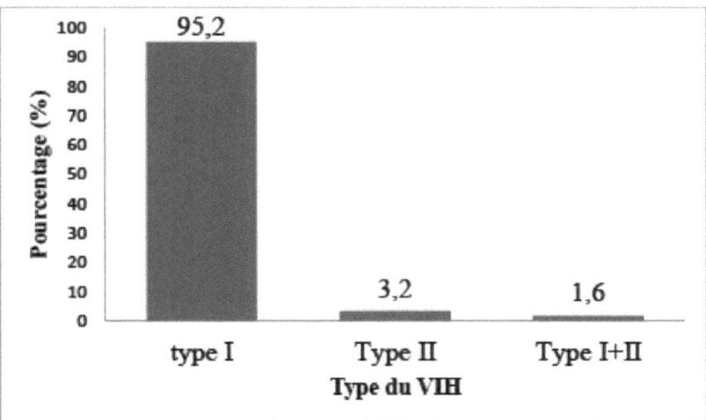


**Figure XV: Breakdown of patients by HIV type**

HIV type I predominated, accounting for 95.2% of cases.

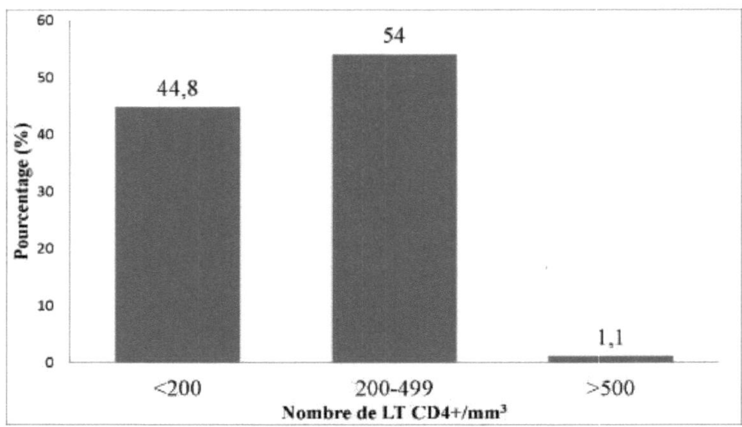


**Figure XVI: Distribution of patients by absolute value**

**CD4+ T lymphocytes**

Patients with severe immunodepression (CD4<200) were estimated to account for 44.8% of cases.

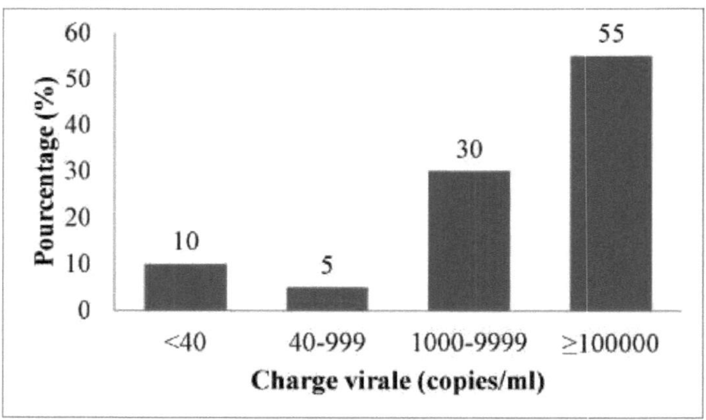


**Figure XVII Breakdown of patients according to viral load (CV)**

Patients had a high viral load in 55% of cases.

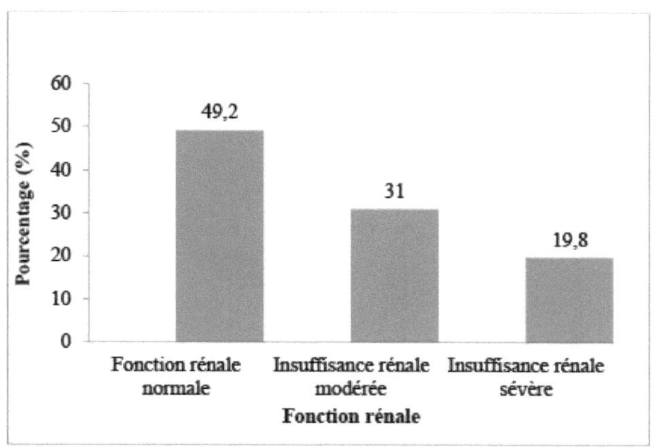


**Figure XVIII Distribution of patients according to renal function**

Patients had normal renal function in 49.2% of cases.

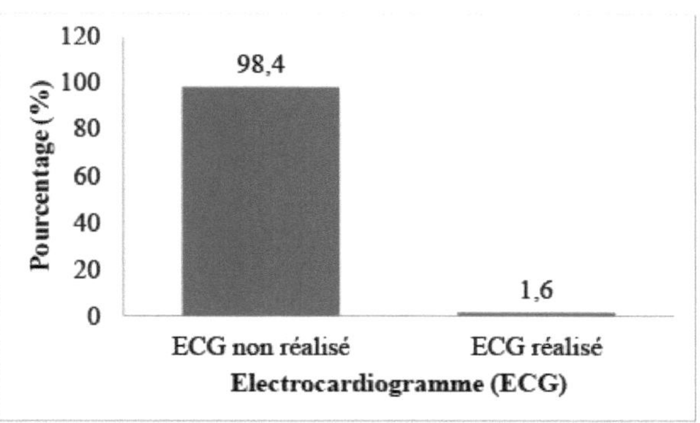


**Electrocardiogram (ECG)**

**Figure XIX : Breakdown of patients according to the ECG performed**

ECGs were not performed in 98.4% of cases. The ECG was normal in the 2 patients who did perform it. Of these 2 patients, one had hyponatremia of 132 mmol/l and hypokalemia of 3.4 mmol/l; the other had hyponatremia of 129 mmol/l. Of the patients who did not have an ECG, 83 (66.9%) had dysnatremia and 50 (40.3%) had dyskalemia.

**IH-1-5-Therapeutic data :**

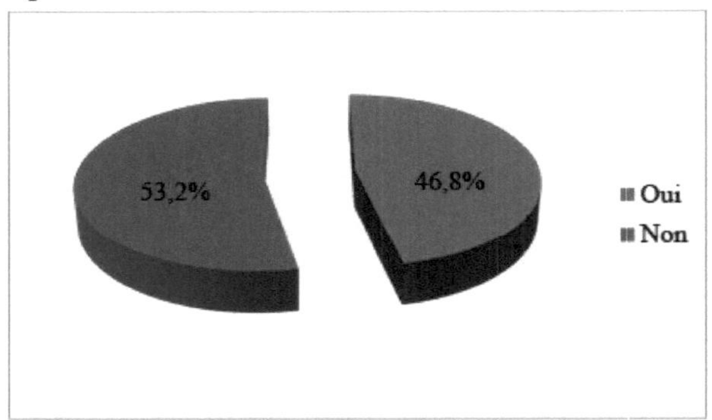


**Figure XX Breakdown of patients by antiretroviral treatment**
Patients were not receiving any ARV treatment in 53.2% of cases.

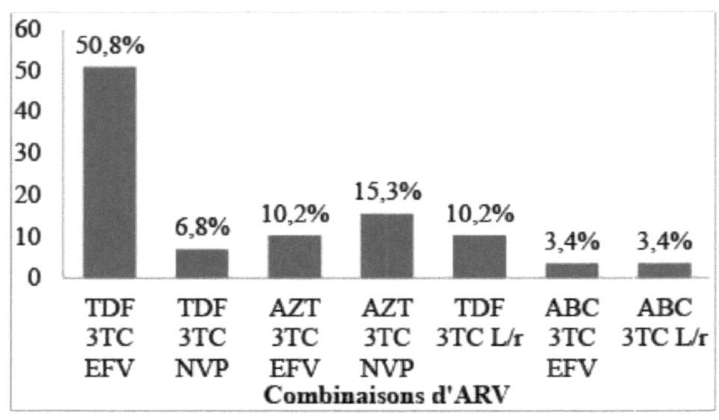


**ARV combinations**

**Figure XXI: Breakdown of patients by ARV combination**
TDF 3TC EFV was the most frequent ARV combination (50.8%).

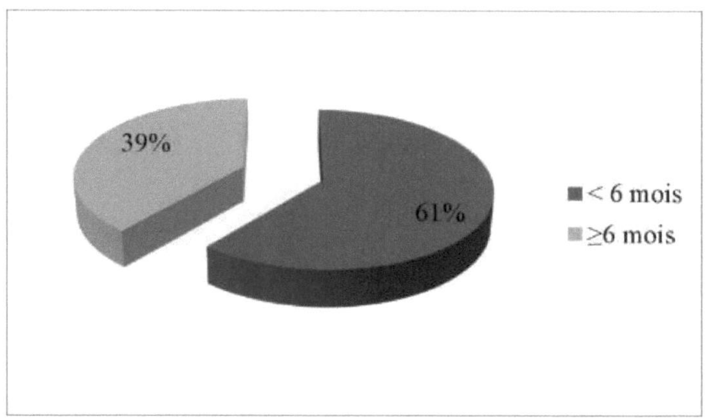


**Figure XXII Breakdown of patients by duration of ART (from initiation)**

Patients had been taking ARVs for less than 6 months in 61% of cases.

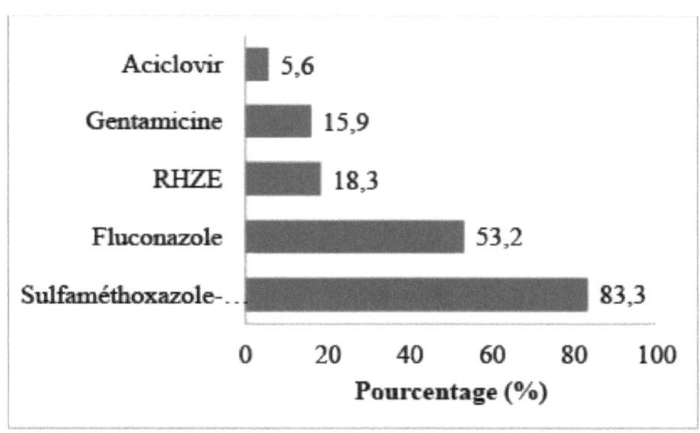


**Figure XXIII Breakdown of patients according to the associated treatment**

Sulfamethoxazole-trimethoprim was taken by 83.3% of patients, followed by fluconazole in 53.2% of cases.

**IH-1-6-Revolution data :**

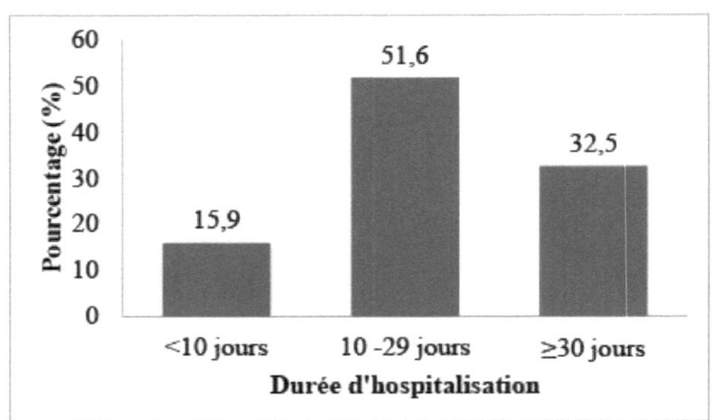


**Figure XXIV Breakdown of patients by length of stay in hospital**

Patients staying between 10 and 30 days predominated, accounting for 57.1% of cases.

The average length of stay was estimated at 25±17 days, with extremes of 1 and 100 days in hospital.

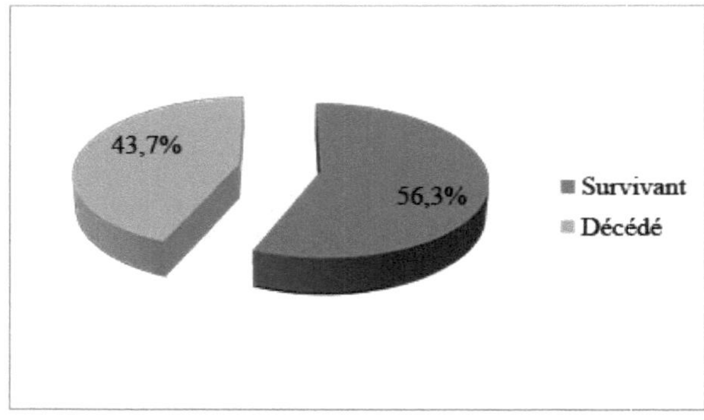


■ Survivor

■ Decede

**Figure XXV Breakdown of patients by outcome**

Hospital mortality is estimated at 43.7%.

**III-2-Analytical study**

**Table VIII: Bivariate analysis of factors associated with death**

| Parameters | Future n (%) | | P |
|---|---|---|---|
| | Survivor | Decede | |
| **Gender** | | | |
| Male | 31(53,4) | 27 (46,6) | 0,544 |
| Female | 40(58,8) | 28(41,2) | |
| **Age** | | | |
| <50 years | 50(58,1) | 36(41,) | 0,552 |

| | | | |
|---|---|---|---|
| > 50 years | 21(52,5) | 19(47,5) | |
| **Natremie** | | | |
| Normalatremia | 28(68,3) | 13(31,7) | 0,161 |
| Hyponatremia | 37(51,4) | 35(48,6) | |
| Hyperatremia | 6(46,2) | 7(53,8) | |
| **Kaliemie** | | | |
| Normal kaliemy | 44(58,7) | 31(41,3) | 0,813 |
| Hypokalemia | 22(52,4) | 20(47,6) | |
| Hyperkalemia | 5(55,6) | 4(44,4) | |
| **Kidney function** | | | |
| <90ml/min | 36(61,0) | 23(39,0) | 0,271 |
| > 90ml/min | 29(50,9) | 28(49,1) | |
| **ARV** | | | |
| Yes | 36(61,0) | 23(39,0) | 0,321 |
| No | 35(52,2) | 32(47,8) | |
| **CD4** | | | |
| <200 | 36(53,7) | 31(46,3) | **0,012** |
| > 200 | 17(85,0) | 3(15,0) | |
| **Dehydration** | | | |
| Yes | 32(46,4) | 37(54,6) | **0,010** |
| No | 39(68,4) | 18(31,6) | |
| **Acute malnutrition** | | | |
| Yes | 40(53,3) | 35(46,7) | 0,095 |
| No | 20(76,9) | 6(23,1) | |
| **Toxoplasmosis cerebral** | | | |
| Yes | 12(36,4) | 21(63,6) | **0,007** |
| No | 59(63,4) | 34(36,6) | |

Mortality was linked to certain factors: the level of immunodepression with

p=0.012; hydration status with p=0.010 and cerebral toxoplasmosis with p=0.007.

The death rate was higher in patients with electrolyte disorders, with p=0.161 for dysnatremia and p=0.813 for dyskaliemia.

**Table IX: Distribution of patients according to status (hydration and nutrition) and natremia**

| State of hydration and nutrition | | Natremia n (%) Normal | Hyponatremia | Hypernatremia | P |
|---|---|---|---|---|---|
| Dehydration | Yes | 24(34,8) | 39(56,5) | 6(8,7) | 0,112 |

| | No | 17(29,8) | 33(57,9) | 7(12,3) | |
|---|---|---|---|---|---|
| Malnutrition acute | Yes | 25(33,3) | 41(54,7) | 9(12,0) | 0,850 |
| | No | 10(38,5) | 15(57,7) | 1(3,8) | |

Dehydrated patients had more dysnatremia (65.2%), as did malnourished patients (66.7%), with p=0.112 and 0.850 respectively.

There was no statistically significant difference between these different states and dysnatremia.

**Table X: Distribution of patients according to digestive signs and natremia**

| **Digestive signs** | | **Natremia n (%)** | | | **P** |
|---|---|---|---|---|---|
| | | **Normal** | **Hyponatremia** | **Hypernatremia** | |
| Diarrhea | Yes | 18(33,3) | 31(57,4) | 5(9,3) | 0,941 |
| | No | 23(31,9) | 41(56,9) | 8(11,1) | |
| Vomiting | Yes | 15(40,5) | 16(43,2) | 6(16,2) | 0,098 |
| | No | 26(29,2) | 56(62,9) | 7(7,9) | |
| Anorexia | Yes | 27(36,0) | 41(54,7) | 7(9,3) | 0,590 |
| | No | 14(27,5) | 31(60,8) | 6(11,8) | |
| Constipation | Yes | 1(50,0) | 1(50,0) | 0(0,0) | 1,000 |
| | No | 40(32,3) | 71(57,3) | 13(10,5) | |

There was no statistically significant difference between digestive signs and dysnatremia.

**Table XI: Distribution of patients according to neurological signs and neatremia**

| **Neurological signs** | | **Natremia n (%)** | | | **P** |
|---|---|---|---|---|---|
| | | **Normal** | **Hyponatremia** | **Hypernatremia** | |
| Depressive syndrome | Yes | 1(100,0) | 0(0,0) 72(57,6) | 0(0,0) | 0,429 |
| | No | 40(32,0) | | 13(10,4) | |
| Disorders of the awareness | Yes | 13(29,5) | 24(54,5) | 7(15,9) | 0,346 |
| | No | 28(34,1) | 48(58,5) | 6(7,3) | |
| Crises convulsive | Yes | 1(9,1) | 9(81,8) | 1(9,1) | 0,185 |
| | No | 40(34,8) | 63(54,8) | 12(10,4) | |
| Delire | Yes | 1(12,5) | 7(87,5) | 0(0,0) | 0,283 |
| | No | 40(33,9) | 65(55,1) | 13(11,0) | |
| Trembling | Yes | 4(40,0) | 6(60,0) | 0(0,0) | 0,792 |
| | No | 37(31,9) | 66(56,9) | 13(11,2) | |
| Deficit neurological motor | Yes | 10(38,5) | 15(57,7) | 1(3,8) | 0,444 |
| | No | 31(31,0) | 57(57,0) | 12(12,0) | |

There was no statistically significant difference between the signs and dysnatremia.

**Table XII: Distribution of patients according to signs of hypertension and neatremia**

| Signs of intracranial hypertension | | Natremia n (%) | | | P |
|---|---|---|---|---|---|
| | | Normal | Hyponatremia | Hypernatremia | 0,600 |
| Cephalees rebelles | Yes | 5(27,8) | 10(55,6) | 3(16,7) | |
| | No | 36(33,3) | 62(57,4) | 10(9,3) | |
| Vomiting incoercible | Yes | 2(28,6) | 4(57,1) | 1(14,3) | 0,864 |
| | No | 39(32,8) | 68(57,1) | 12(10,1) | |

There was no statistically significant difference between the signs of intracranial hypertension found in the patients and the dysnatremia.

**Table XIII: Distribution of patients according to muscular signs striae and neatremia**

| Muscular signs striae | | Natremia n (%) | | | P |
|---|---|---|---|---|---|
| | | Normal | Hyponatremia | Hypernatremia | |
| Fatigability | Yes | 9(42,9) | 10(47,6) | 2(9,5) | 0,526 |
| | No | 32(30,5) | 62(59,0) | 11(10,5) | |
| Hypotonia muscular | Yes | 3(42,9) | 4(57,1) | 0(0,0) | 0,864 |
| | No | 38(31,9) | 68(57,1) | 13(10,9) | |

There was no statistically significant difference between muscle striae and dysnatremia.

**Table XIV: Breakdown of patients by diagnostic pathology and natremia**

| Diagnosed diseases | | Natremia n (%) | | | P |
|---|---|---|---|---|---|
| | | Normal | Hyponatremia | Hypernatremia | |
| Tuberculosis | Yes | 5(20,0) | 20(80,0) | 0(0,0) | **0,018** |
| | No | 36(35,6) | 52(51,5) | 13(12,9) | |
| Pneumopathy bacterial non tuberculous | Yes | 7(36,8) | 10(52,6) | 2(10,5) | 0,933 |
| | No | 34(31,8) | 62(57,9) | 11(10,3) | |
| Toxoplasmosis cerebral | Yes | 14(42,4) | 16(48,5) | 3(9,1) | 0,375 |
| | No | 27(29,0) | 56(60,2) | 10(10,8) | |
| Simple malaria | Yes | 2(25,0) | 6(75,0) | 0(0,0) | 0,649 |
| | No | 39(33,1) | 66(55,9) | 13(11,0) | |
| Severe malaria | Yes | 3(20,0) | 10(66,7) | 2(13,3) | 0,599 |
| | No | 38(34,2) | 62(55,9) | 11(9,9) | |
| Candidiasis oral | Yes | 24(34,8) | 37(53,6) | 8(11,6) | 0,668 |
| | No | 17(29,8) | 35(61,4) | 5(8,8) | |

| | | | | | |
|---|---|---|---|---|---|
| Isosporosis | Yes | 2(66,7) | 1(33,3) | 0(0,0) | 0,495 |
| | No | 39(31,7) | 71(57,7) | 13(10,6) | |
| Infections lower urinary tract | Yes | 9(45,0) | 10(50,0) | 1(5,0) | 0,474 |
| | No | 32(30,2) | 62(58,5) | 12(11,3) | |
| Diarrhoea bacterial and/or parasites | Yes | 6(35,3) | 10(58,8) | 1(5,9) | 1,000 |
| | No | 35(32,1) | 62(56,9) | 12(11,0) | |

Among the pathologies diagnosed, there was a statistically significant difference between tuberculosis and dysnatremia (p=0.018).

**Table XV: Distribution of patients according to renal function and natremia**

| Renal function | Natremia n (%) Normal | Hyponatremia | Hypernatremia | P |
|---|---|---|---|---|
| Kidney function | 19(33,3) | 31(54,4) | 7(12,3) | 0,996 |
| Moderate renal failure | 11(30,6) | 21(58,3) | 4(11,1) | |
| Renal insufficiency severe | 7 (30,6) | 14 (60,9) | 2 (8,7) | |

There was no statistically significant difference between patients' renal function and dysnatremia.

**Table XVI: Distribution of patients according to treatment and natremia**

| Type of treatment | | Natremia n (%) | | | P |
|---|---|---|---|---|---|
| | | Normal | Hyponatremia | Hypernatremia | |
| RDRV | Yes | 21(35,6) | 34(57,6) | 4(6,8) | 0,434 |
| | No | 20(29,9) | 38(56,7) | 9(13,4) | |
| Sulfamethoxazole-Trimethoprime | Yes | 37(35,2) | 59(56,2) | 9(8,6) | 0,173 |
| | No | 4(20,0) | 12(60,0) | 4(20,0) | |
| Fluconazole | Yes | 26(38,8) | 33(49,3) | 8(11,9) | 0,161 |
| | No | 15(25,4) | 39(66,1) | 5(8,5) | |
| acyclovir | Yes | 2(28,6)) | 3(42,9) | 2(28,6) | 0,271 |
| | No | 39(32,8) | 69(58,0) | 11(9,2) | |
| RHZE | Yes | 4(17,4) | 19(82,6) | 0(0,0) | **0,016** |
| | No | 37(35,9) | 53(51,5) | 13(12,6) | |
| Gentamicin | Yes | 9(45,0) | 10(50,0) | 1(5,0) | 0,474 |
| | No | 32(30,2) | 62(58,5) | 12(11,3) | |

Among the drugs taken by patients, there was a statistically significant difference between anti-tuberculosis drugs (RHZE) and dysnatremia (p=0.016).

**Table XVII: Distribution of patients according to state (of hydration and of nutrition) and kaliemie**

| Conditions (hydration | Normal | Kaliemie n (%) | P |
|---|---|---|---|

| and nutrition) | | | Hypokalemia | Hyperkalemia | |
|---|---|---|---|---|---|
| Dehydration | Yes | 38(55,1) | 28(40,6) | 3(4,3) | 0,112 |
| | No | 37(64,9) | 14(24,6) | 6(10,5) | |
| Malnutrition acute | Yes | 36(48,0) | 34(45,3%) | 5(6,7%) | **0,023** |
| | No | 21(80,8) | 3(11,5) | 2(7,7) | |

There was a statistically significant difference between nutritional status and dyskalaemia (p=0.023).

**Table XVIII: Distribution of patients according to digestive signs and kaliemy**

| Digestive signs | | Kaliemie n (%) | | | P |
|---|---|---|---|---|---|
| | | Normal | Hypokalemia | Hyperkalemia | |
| Diarrhea | Yes | 27(50,0) | 25(46,3) | 2(3,7) | **0,023** |
| | No | 48(66,7) | 17(23,6) | 7(9,7) | |
| Vomiting | Yes | 21(56,8) | 14(37,8) | 2(5,4) | 0,779 |
| | No | 54(60,7) | 28(31,5) | 7(7,9) | |
| Anorexia | Yes | 45(60,0) | 25(33,3) | 5(6,7) | 1,000 |
| | No | 30(58,8) | 17(33,3) | 4(7,8) | |
| Constipation | Yes | 2(100,0) | 0(0,0) | 0(0,0) | 0,600 |
| | No | 73(58,9) | 42(33,9) | 9(7,3) | |

Among the digestive signs found in patients, there was a statistically significant association between diarrhoea and the occurrence of dyskalaemia (p=0.023).

**Table XIX: Distribution of patients according to neurological signs and kalemia**

| Neurological signs | | Kaliemie n (%) | | | P |
|---|---|---|---|---|---|
| | | Normal | Hypokalemia | Hyperkalemia | 0,405 |
| Depressive syndrome | Yes | 0(0,0) | 1(100,0) | 0(0,0) | |
| | No | 75(60,0) | 41(32,8) | 9(7,2) | |
| Disorders of the awareness | Yes | 31(70,5) | 9(20,5) | 4(9,1) | 0,075 |
| | No | 44(53,7) | 33(40,2) | 5(6,1) | |
| Crises convulsive | Yes | 7(63,6) | 3(27,3) | 1(9,1) | 0,891 |
| | No | 68(59,1) | 39(33,9) | 8(7,0) | |
| Delire | Yes | 7(87,5) | 1(12,5) | 0(0,0) | 0,389 |
| | No | 68(57,6) | 41(34,7) | 9(7,6) | |
| Trembling | Yes | 6(60,0) | 2(20,0) | 2(20,0) | 0,184 |
| | No | 69(59,5) | 40(34,5) | 7(6,0) | |
| Deficit neurological | Yes | 20(76,9) | 5(19,2) | 1(3,8) | 0,132 |
| | No | 55(55,0) | 37(37,0) | 8(8,0) | |

motor

There was no statistically significant association between neurological signs in patients and dyskalemia.

**Table XX: Distribution of patients according to signs of intracranial hypertension and kalemia**

| Signs of hypertension intracranial | | Kaliemia n (%) Normal | Hypokaliemia | Hyperkaliemia | P |
|---|---|---|---|---|---|
| Cephalees rebelles | Yes | 15(83,3) | 3(16,7) | 0(0,0) | 0,096 |
| | No | 60(55,6) | 39(36,1) | 9(8,3) | |
| Vomiting incoercible | Yes | 6(85,7) | 1(14,3) | 0(0,0) | 0,547 |
| | No | 69(58,0) | 41(34,5) | 9(7,6) | |

There was no statistically significant association between signs of intracranial hypertension in patients and dyskalemia.

**Table XXI: Distribution of patients according to muscular signs striae and kaliemy**

| Muscular signs striae | | Kaliemie n (%) | | | P |
|---|---|---|---|---|---|
| | | **Normal** | **Hypokalemia** | **Hyperkalemia** | |
| Fatigability | Yes | 10(47,6) | 9(42,9) | 2(9,5) | 0,442 |
| | No | 65(61,9) | 33(31,4) | 7(6,7) | |
| Hypotonia muscular | Yes | 5(71,4) | 2(28,6) | 0(0,0) | 1,000 |
| | No | 70(58,8) | 40(33,6) | 9(7,6) | |

There was no statistically significant association between the muscle striae signs found in patients and dyskalaemia.

**Table XXII: Breakdown of patients by diagnosed pathologies and kaliemia**

| | | Kaliemie n (%) | | | P |
|---|---|---|---|---|---|
| **Diagnosed diseases** | | **Normal** | **Hypokalemia** | **Hyperkalemia** | |
| Tuberculosis | Yes | 12(48,0) | 11(44,0) | 2(8,0) | 0,402 |
| | No | 63(62,4) | 31(30,7) | 7(6,9) | |
| Pneumopathy bacterial non tuberculous | Yes | 14(73,7) | 4(21,1) | 1(5,3) | 0,450 |
| | No | 61(57,0) | 38(35,5) | 8(7,5) | |
| Toxoplasmosis cerebral | Yes | 28(84,8) | 5(15,2) | 0(0,0) | **0,002** |
| | No | 47(50,5) | 37(39,8) | 9(9,7) | |
| Simple malaria | Yes | 3(37,5) | 5(62,5) | 0(0,0) | 0,208 |
| | No | 72(61,0) | 37(31,4) | 9(7,6) | |
| Severe malaria | Yes | 9(60,0) | 5(33,3) | 1(6,7) | 1,000 |
| | No | 66(59,5) | 37(33,3) | 8(7,2) | |

| | | | | | |
|---|---|---|---|---|---|
| Oral candidiasis | Yes | 34(49,3) | 31(44,9) | 4(5,8) | **0,008** |
| | No | 41(71,9) | 11(19,3) | 5(8,8) | |
| Isosporosis | Yes | 1(33,3) | 1(33,3) | 1(33,3) | 0,236 |
| | No | 74(60,2) | 41(33,3) | 8(6,5) | |
| Infections lower urinary tract | Yes | 11(55,0) | 7(35,0) | 2(10,0) | 0,736 |
| | No | 64(60,4) | 35(33,0) | 7(6,6%) | |
| Diarrhoea bacterial and/or parasitic | Yes | 9(52,9) | 7(41,2) | 1(5,9) | 0,834 |
| | No | 66(60,6) | 35(32,1) | 8(7,3) | |

Among the pathologies diagnosed, there was a statistically significant difference between cerebral toxoplasmosis and dyskalaemia (p=0.002), and between oral candidiasis and dyskalaemia (p=0.008).

**Table XXIII: Distribution of patients according to renal function and kalemia**

| **Renal function** | **Kalemia n (%)P Normal** | **Hypokalemia** | **Hyperkalemia** | |
|---|---|---|---|---|
| Normal kidney function | 32(56,1) | 19 (33,3) | 6 (10,5) | 0,872 |
| Moderate renal failure | 24(66,7) | 10 (27,8) | 2 (5,5) | |
| Renal insufficiency severe | 16(69,6) | 7 (30,4) | 0 (0,0) | |

There was no statistically significant difference between patients' renal function and dyskalemia.

**Table XXIV: Distribution of patients according to treatment and kaliemia**

| **Type of treatment** | | **Kaliemia n (%)P Normal** | **Hypokalemia** | **Hyperkalemia** | |
|---|---|---|---|---|---|
| RDRV | Yes | 29(49,2) | 27(45,8) | 3(5,1) | **0,020** |
| | No | 46(68,7) | 15(22,4) | 6(9,0) | |
| Sulfamethoxazole-Trimethoprime | Yes | 66(62,9) | 33(31,4) | 6(5,7) | 0,163 |
| | No | 9 (45,0) | 8(40,0) | 3(15,0) | |
| Fluconazole | Yes | 34(50,7) | 29(43,3) | 4(6,0) | **0,041** |
| | No | 41(69,5) | 13(22,0) | 5(8,5) | |
| acyclovir | Yes | 4(57,1) | 3(42,9) | 0(0,0) | 0,824 |
| | No | 71(59,7) | 39(32,8) | 9(7,6) | |
| RHZE | Yes | 10(43,5) | 11(47,8) | 2(8,7) | 0,190 |
| | No | 65(63,1) | 31(30,1) | 7(6,8) | |
| Gentamicin | Yes | 13(65,0) | 6(30,0) | 1(5,0) | 0,925 |
| | No | 62(58,5) | 36(34,0) | 8(7,5) | |

There was a statistically significant difference between dyskalemia and certain drugs taken by patients: ARVs (p=0.020) and fluconazole (p=0.041).

**Table XXV: Distribution of patients according to renal function and antiretroviral treatment**

| | Renal function n (%) | | | P |
|---|---|---|---|---|
| | Renal function normal | Insufficiency moderate kidney disease | Insufficiency severe renal disease | 0.811 |
| **ART** Yes | 27(51.9) | 15(28.9) | 10 (19.2) | |
| No | 30(46.9) | 21(32.8) | 13 (20.3) | |

In patients who had not received any ARV treatment, renal failure was moderate in 32.8% and severe in 20.3% of cases (p=0.811).

## 4 A DISCUSSION

In the world and in Africa, particularly in Mali, very few studies have been devoted to electrolyte disorders in the hospital environment, particularly in people living with HIV. The originality of our study lies in this. It was conducted retrospectively over a period of six years in the infectious diseases department of the Point G University Hospital. The aim of the study was to describe electrolyte disorders in HIV-infected patients in a hospital setting. As with any retrospective study, our work has its limitations, in particular the inability to use the files due to lack of data and the lack of follow-up of patients discharged from hospital. Despite these limitations, the results of our study give rise to the following discussion:

### IV-1-Epidemiology :

One hundred and twenty-six hospital records collected over 6 years met our inclusion criteria. This number is higher than that of Peter et al who collected 81 cases at Woodhull Hospital in New York over 4 years [57].

### IV-2-Social and demographic characteristics :

Patients ranged in age from 22 to 70, with an average age of 43. The 28-37 age group was the most represented with 27% and a sex ratio of 0.85. Our results are consistent with those of Emejulu et al [3] with respect to age extremes and sex predominance, whereas they differ from those of Peter et al [57] who noted a male predominance.

### IV-3-Clinical data :

The reasons for hospitalisation, in order of frequency, were deterioration in general condition (59.5%), followed by chronic diarrhoea (23.8%) and long-term fever (20.6%).

Diarrhoea and fever are cited in the literature as underlying causes of electrolyte disorders in PLHIV [4, 62,63].

Patients were polypneic in 76% of cases, febrile in 46% and hypovolemic in 50%. All these factors have been found in the literature to favour electrolyte disorders, particularly hyponatremia in PLWHA [4, 63].

Patients were dehydrated in 54.8% of cases and malnourished in 74.2%.

Dehydrated patients had more dysnatremia (65.2%), as did malnourished patients (66.7%), with p=0.112 and 0.850 respectively.

There was no statistically significant difference between these different states and dysnatremia.

This can be explained by the leakage of electrolytes during clinical situations that are conducive to dehydration and malnutrition, in particular episodes of uncontrollable vomiting, profuse diarrhoea, fever and polypnoea.

The proportion of dyskalemia was higher in dehydrated patients (hypokalemia=40.6%; hyperkalemia=4.3%) with p=0.112.

There was a statistically significant difference between nutritional status and dyskalaemia (p=0.023). This result is supported by another in our study, namely the existence of a statistically significant link between diarrhoea and dyskalaemia (p=0.023).

These results show that acute malnutrition and diarrhoea are favourable factors for electrolyte disorders (dyskalaemia) in HIV-infected patients.

The clinical signs in order of frequency were anorexia (59.5%), diarrhoea (42.9%), disturbed consciousness (34.9%) and vomiting (29.4%).

There was no statistically significant difference between the patients' clinical signs and dysnatremia. These results are consistent with those of the clinical review of the literature on the treatment of electrolyte disorders in adult intensive care unit patients by Michael et al, who found that the clinical signs associated with hyponatremia were often non-specific [55].

The most frequently diagnosed pathologies were oral candidiasis (54.8%), followed by cerebral toxoplasmosis (26.2%) and all forms of tuberculosis (19.8%).

Among the pathologies diagnosed, there was a statistically significant difference between tuberculosis and dysnatremia (p=0.018); similarly between cerebral toxoplasmosis and dyskalaemia (p=0.002); and between oral candidiasis and dyskalaemia (p=0.008).

Our patients were divided into clinical stages II, III and IV, with stage IV predominating (54%).

Given that tuberculosis and cerebral toxoplasmosis are events classifying as AIDS and oral candidiasis classifies the patient as stage II, these results are in line with those of Eshiet et al [64] who found a statistically significant difference between natremia, kalemia, chloremia and the different stages of HIV infection in Ekpoma, Nigeria.

They are also in line with those of Ansger (2007) [65] and Ross et al (2004) [66] who observed that HIV infection can lead to electrolyte and acid-base disorders and pathologies directly related to the different stages of the infection.

**IV-4-Biological data :**

In this study, the electrolyte disorders found were hyponatremia (41.2%), hypokalemia (12.7%), hypematremia (7.8%), hyperkalemia (2.9%) and associated disorders (35.3%). Among the cases of hyponatremia, 50% were depletion hyponatremia, 50% dilution hyponatremia and no inflation hyponatremia.

These results differ from those obtained by Onwuliri in 2004, who did not find any electrolyte disorders in HIV-infected patients newly undergoing treatment at

Jos in Nigeria [67]. The difference could be due to the stage of infection of the patients or to their idiosyncrasy varying from one centre to another [3]. While they are consistent with some earlier data. Peter (1991) observed 28.4% hyponatremia, 17.3% hypokalemia and 4.9% hyperkalemia without renal failure in a group of Latino and African-American patients infected with HIV [57]. Emejulu (2011) found 47.5% hypematremia, 22.5% hyponatremia and 32.5% hypokalemia in asymptomatic HIV-infected patients in Nigeria [3]. This reinforces the idea that acute or chronic renal dysfunction associated with HIV infection and nephropathy occur predominantly in African-American patients and generally in black patients [3, 68]. Our study supports this hypothesis because 32.8% of our ARV-naïve patients had moderate renal failure and 20.3% had severe renal failure (p=0.811).

The syndrome of inappropriate anti-diuretic hormone secretion (SIADH) is the second most common cause of hyponatremia after hypovolemia in HIV-infected patients [63]. In most cases, it results either from the infection or from cancer of the central nervous system or respiratory system [63].

Hypematremia occurs when water loss far exceeds water intake.

The causes of water loss in HIV-infected patients are, on the one hand, manifestations of opportunistic infections or tumours (fever, hypersudation, polypnoea, diarrhoea) and, on the other hand, nephrogenic diabetic insipidus due to OIs or tumours or induced by drugs used in the treatment of OIs, in particular foscarnet, rifampicin and amphotericin B [63].

These reasons could explain the statistically significant link observed in our study between dysnatremia and tuberculosis (p=0.018) on the one hand, and its treatment (p=0.016) on the other.

The statistically significant association observed between dyskalaemia and cerebral toxoplasmosis (p=0.002); oral candidiasis (p=0.008); diarrhoea (p=0.023); nutritional status (p=0.023); and ARV treatment (p=0.020) is explained by the causes of dyskalaemia mentioned in the literature reviews by Musso et al [4]; Mark et al [63]. In these reviews, hypokalemia results from :

- or an increase in gastrointestinal potassium loss (diarrhoea of infectious or tumour origin, or due to enteropathy associated with AIDS);
- or by an increase in renal potassium leakage (hyperaldosteronism secondary to hypovolemia induced by incoercible vomiting or direct nephrotoxicity of certain drugs such as amphotericin B, aminoglycosides, tenofovir, zidovudine or interstitial nephritis secondary to certain antibiotics, particularly sulphonamides and cephalosporins);
- at the end or by an inadequate intake of potassium (anorexia, undernourishment, etc.) [4].

In addition, encephalic involvement during cerebral toxoplasmosis is a cause of transfer hypokalemia [52].

As for the hyperkalemia, it is thought to be due to :

- or a reduction in urinary potassium excretion by drugs such as trimethoprim in the case of renal insufficiency or suprarenal insufficiency or hypoaldosteronism;
- or an increase in potassium transfer to the extracellular medium [4].

HIV type I predominated with 95.2% of cases. This result is similar to that of Sissoko [45] who found a predominance of HIV-1 (96%).

Patients with severe immunodepression (CD4<200) were estimated at 44.8% of cases. This is significantly lower than the 63.3% recorded by Sissoko [45] as the proportion of patients with a CD4 count<200.

**IV-5-Therapeutic treatment :**

Patients were ART-naïve in 53.2% of cases. This was the case in the Emejulu study in Nigeria [3], in which 100% of patients were newly diagnosed with HIV and not initiated on ARVs.

TDF 3TC EFV was the most frequent ARV regimen (50.8%). This can be explained by the national guidelines for the management of PLHIV in Mali, which recommend this combination as the preferred regimen in cases of HIV-1 infection.

Sulfamethoxazole-trimethoprim was taken by 83.3% of patients, followed by fluconazole in 53.2% of cases. These results concur with those of Sissoko [45] regarding the use of Sulfamethoxazole-Trimethoprim, which represented 86.7% of combined treatments.

**IV-6-Evolution :**

Patients staying between 10 and 30 days predominated, accounting for 57.1% of cases. The average length of stay was estimated at 25±17 days, with extremes of 1 and 100 days in hospital. This long hospital stay would seem to put patients with severe immunodepression at greater risk of nosocomial infections.

Hospital mortality was estimated at 43.7%. The death rate was higher in patients with electrolyte disorders, with p=0.161 for dysnatremia and p=0.813 for dyskaliemia.

Mortality was related to the level of immunodepression (p=0.012), hydration status (p=0.010) and cerebral toxoplasmosis (p=0.007). The significant association of these 3 parameters with death could largely explain the high mortality rate recorded in our study.

## 5 CONCLUSION AND RECOMMENDATIONS

Electrolyte disorders are common in patients with HIV/AIDS. Efficient management of these disorders requires multidisciplinary involvement (infectiologists, biologists, nephrologists and resuscitators).

This leads us to make a number of recommendations.

**To the administrative health authorities:**

- supply the Point G University Hospital laboratory with reagents for measuring ions in various body fluids on a regular basis,
- reduce the cost of ionograms,
- make the different presentations of electrolytes and medical consumables available at the Point G hospital pharmacy,
- equip each department with an electrocardiograph.

**Medical staff:**

- regularly monitor the hydration and nutritional status of hospitalised patients,
- systematic weekly screening for electrolyte disorders in hospitalised patients,
- request an electrocardiogram in the event of any abnormality in the blood ionogram,
- facilitate multidisciplinary management of hospitalised patients.

**Paramedical staff:**

- scrupulously observe the rules for taking blood samples,
- correctly carrying out the therapeutic protocol for hospitalised patients.

**To patients and parents:**

- Comply on time with medical prescriptions, check-ups for electrolyte disorders and monitoring of treatment,
- follow medical advice and observe the instructions for taking biological samples.

## REFERENCES

1-Leport C, Longuet P, Gervais A and Vilde JL. Clinical manifestations of human immunodeficiency virus infection. Encycl Med Chir (Editions Scientifiques et Medicales Elsevier SAS, Paris, all rights reserved), Maladies infectieuses, 8-050-B-10, 2002, 20 p.

2-Bouroignie J J. Renal complications of human immunodeficiency virus type 1. Kidney int 1990 ;37 :1571-84.

3-Emejulu AA, Onwuliri VA. and Ojiako OA. Electrolyte Abnormalities and Renal Impairment in Asymptomatic HIV-infected Patients in Owerri, South Eastern Nigeria. Australian Journal of Basic and Applied Sciences. 2011; 5(3): 257-60.

4-Musso CG, Belloso WH, Glassock RJ. Water, electrolytes, and acid-base alterations in human immunodeficiency virus infected patients. World J Nephrol. 2016; 5(1): 33-42.

5- Hsu DC, Sereti I, Ananworanich J. Serious Non-AIDS events: Immunopathogenesis and interventional strategies. AIDS Res Ther 2013; 10: 29 [PMID: 24330529 DOI: 10.1186/1742-6405-10-29]

6- Serrano-Villar S, Perez-EHas MJ, Dronda F et al.Increased risk of serious non- AIDS-related events in HIV-infected subjects on antiretroviral therapy associated with a low CD4/CD8 ratio. PLoS One 2014; 9: e85798 [PMID: 24497929 DOI: 10.1371/journal.pone.0085798]

7- Fux CA, Simcock M, Wolbers M et al. Tenofovir use is associated with a reduction in calculated glomerular filtration rates in the Swiss HIV Cohort Study. Antivir Ther 2007; 12: 1165-73. [PMID: 18240857]

8- Cooper RD, Wiebe N, Smith N et al. Systematic review and meta-analysis: renal safety of tenofovir disoproxil fumarate in HIV-infected patients. Clin Infect Dis 2010; 51: 496-505. [PMID: 20673002 DOI: 10.1086/655681]

9- Labarga P, Barreiro P, Martin-Carbonero L et al. Kidney tubular abnormalities in the absence of impaired glomerular function in HIV patients treated with tenofovir. AIDS 2009; 23: 689-96. [PMID: 19262355 DOI: 10.1097/ QAD.0b013e3283262a64]

10-Mignon F, Michel C, Albert C, Viron B. Problemes nephrologiques au cours de l'infection par le virus de l'immunodeficience humaine. Editions techniques. Encycl. Med. Chir (Paris-France). Nephrology-Urology 18066 L10, 1992,4p

11- Maggi P, Montinaro V, Mussini C et al. Novel antiretroviral drugs and renal function monitoring of HIV patients. AIDS Rev 2014; 16: 144-51. [PMID: 25102336]

12- Estrella MM, Fine DM. Screening for chronic kidney disease in HIV-infected patients. Adv Chronic Kidney Dis 2010; 17: 26-35. [PMID: 20005486

DOI: 10.1053/j.ackd.2009.07.014]
13-Fomo KD. Etat nutritionnel et tolerance aux antiretroviraux chez les personnes vivant avec le VIH suivies au service des maladies infectieuses du CHU Point G de Bamako. [These]. Medecine : Bamako ; 2014. p101.
14-WHO | HIV/AIDS [Internet]. [cite 13 jan 2014]. Available from: http://who.int/features/qa/71/fr/index.html
15-History of hiv [Internet]. [cited 16 Jan 2014]; [3pages]. Available from: http://pvsq.org/articles/historique.pdf
16-Escort.8. The variability of HIV, cont [Internet]. [cited 23 Jan 2014]. Available from:
http://www.itg.be/internet/elearning/written_lecture_fr/8_la_variabilit_du_vih_cont1.html
17- Sogoba D. Contribution a l'etude epidemio-clinique du SIDA au service des maladies infectieuses de l'hopital du Point " G ", Bamako, Mali. [These]. Medecine : Bamako ; 2005. p85.
18- Immunology-AIDS. The structure of HIV [Internet]. 14/02/2006 [cite 22 janv 2014]. Available from: http://acces.ens-lyon.fr/biotic/immuno/html/strucvih.htm
19- Gentillini M, Duflo JC. Sida tropical. Medecine tropicale, 1986: 401-13.
20- Brucker G, Tubiana R. Prevention des risques professionnels et regles de desinfection. Doin VIH edition 2011. 839 p.
21- CMIT. HIV infection and AIDS. In E. PILLY: Vivactis Plus Ed ; 2010 : p3689.
22-Laporte A, Lot F. Epidemiology: current situation and trends. Doin VIH edition 2011. 839 p.
23- Caumes E. Dermatological manifestations. Doin VIH edition 2011. 839 p.
24- Connor EM, Sperling RS, Gelber R. Reduction of maternal-infant transmission of human immunodeficiency virus type 1 with Zidovudine treatment N Engl J Med 1994; 331:1175-80.
25-UNAIDS. Global report. UNAIDS report on the global AIDS epidemic/2017 [Internet]. [cited 29 Aug 2017]. Available from: http://aidsinfo.unaids.org/
26-DNSI-CPS/ Ministry of Health. Enquete demographique et de sante Mali (EDNSM IV). Bamako: ministere de la sante, 2006; 497 p.
27-Leport C, Longuet P, Lacassin F, Vilde JL. Manifestations cliniques et therapeutiques de l'infection par le VIH. Encyclopedie Medico-chirurgicale (Elsevier, Paris). Maladies infectieuses, 8-050-B-10, 1996, 16 p.
28-Picard C, Desforges L. Biological diagnostics for HIV. An Dermatol Veneriol. 1989 ;9 : 671-4.
29-Cockerell CJ, Friedman- Kien AE. Cutaneous signs of HIV infection. In:

BRODER S, MERIGNAN TC JR, BOLOGNESI D, eds. Text book of AIDS. medicine. Baltimore: Williams and Wilkins; 1994;507-24.
30-Costner M, Cockerell CJ. The Changing spectrum of the cutaneous manifestations of HIV disease. Archdermatol1994;130: 521-2.
31-Hira SK, Wadhaman D, Kamanga J. Cutaneous manifestations of human immunodeficiency virus in Lusaka. Zambia: J AmAcadDermatol 1988;19: 4517.
32-Tschaler E, Bergstresser PR, Stingl G. HIV related Skin diseases Lancet 1996;N(348): 659-63.
33-Colebunders R, Francis H, Mannjm, Bila K M, Izaley A, Lkimputu L. Persistent diarrhea, strongly associated with HIV infection in KinshasaZaire. An J Gastro Enterol 1987;82: 859-64.
34-Wallace J, Hansen N, Lavange L, al. Respiratory diseases trends in the pulmonary complications of HIV infection study cohort. An J Respire Crit CareMed 1997;155: 72-80.
35-Myers G, Mac IK, Korber B. The emergence of simian/human immunodeficiency viruses. AIDS Res Hun Retrovir 1992;8:373-85.
36- Arthur JMC. Neurologic manifestations of AIDS.Medicine1987; 66: 407-37.
37-Simpson DM, Berger JR. Neurologic manifestations of HIV infection. Med Clin North An 1996; 80:1363-94.
38-Datry A. Digestive candidiasis and HIV infection. Actualites cliniques et therapeutiques. J Mycol Med 1992 ;2 (Suppl 1) : 5-14.
39-Ott M, Lembcke B, Fischer H. Early changes of Body composition I human immunodeficiency virus. Infected patients: Tetrapolar body impedanceanalysisindicatessignificant malnutrition. An J Clin Nutr 1993;57:15-9.
40-Scandden DT. The clinical applications of colony stimulating factors in acquired immunodeficiency syndrome.Seminhematol1992;29 (suppl3):33-7.
41-Cooper DA, Gatell J M, Kroon S et al:Zidovudine in persons with asymptomatic HIV infection and CD 4 + cell counts greater than 400 per cubic millimeter. N Engl J Med 1993 ;329:297-303.
42-Naheed A. Kidney Involvement in HIV Infection. Dr. Eugenia Barros (Ed.) 2011; 336:91-116. Available from: http://www.intechopen.com/books/hiv-infection-impact-awareness-and-social-implications-of-living-withhiv-aids/kidney-involvement-in-hiv-infection
43-Choi et al. Long-term clinical consequences of acute kidney injury in the HIV- infected. Kidney Int. 2010 Sep; 78 (5):478-85.
44-Choi et al: HIV-infected persons continue to lose kidney function despite successful antiretroviral therapy. AIDS 23(16):2143-2149(2009).
45-Sissoko M. Les complications renales au cours du VIH et du traitement par

les ARV a l'hopital du Point G. [These]. Medecine : Bamako ; 2004. p105.
46-.Cellule de coordination du comite sectoriel de lutte contre le SIDA. Politique et protocole de prise en charge antiretrovirale du VIH et SIDA 2016. Bamako; p197.
47- Eholie PS, Girard P, Bissagnene E, editors. Memento therapeutique du VIH/SIDA en Afrique 2017. 3eme ed. Montrouge: John Libbey Eurotext; 2017. 260 p.
48-ESTHER. Goree Recommendations 2001-Initiative Internationale: "place des antiretroviraux dans la prise en charge des personnes infectees par le VIH en Afrique". Developpement et sante 2002 ;162: 15-8.
49-Ould MA. Etude des apports hydrolytiques au cours de l'insuffisance renale chronique dans le service de nephrologie de l'hopital national du Point G. . [These]. Medecine : Bamako ; 2006. p97.
50- Ahuja TS, Agraharkar M. Renal Complications of the Human Immunodeficiency Virus Infection. Saudi J Kidney Dis Transpl 2000;11:1-12.
51- EMC - Medecine d'urgence 2007:1-24 [Article 25-010-D-20].
52-Ebongue LRS. Desordres hydrolytiques chez les patients cerebroleses dans le service de reanimation du CHU Gabriel TOURE . [These]. Medecine : Bamako ; 2016. p107.
53-Medecin des hopitaux-Praticien hospitalier ; Urgences medico-chirurgicales et judiciaires, SMUR ; Hotel- Dieu- Cochin (Paris) ; Universites Paris Descartes Cree : le 21/11/2008 Mis a jour : le 24/03/2010. www.ocp.fr
54-Groupe BiopyreneesLab. Sampling manual MQ MU PRE 001 Version 2. Updated: 24/12/2014. www.biopyrenees.fr.
55- Michael DK et al. Treatment of electrolyte disorders in adult patients in the intensive care unit. Am J Health-Syst Pharm-Vol 62 Aug 15, 2005 p1663-82.
56- Fourcade J. Potassium disorders. Faculte de Medecine Montpellier- Nimes. Nephrology ECN 219 May 2006.
57- Peter SA. Electrolyte disorders and renal dysfunction in acquired immunodeficiency syndrome patients. J Natl Med Assoc 1991;83:889-91. Back to cited text no. 57 [PUBMED].
58- Marks JB. Endocrine manifestations of human immunodeficiency virus (HIV) infection. Am J Med Sci 1991;302:110-7. Back to cited text no. 59 [PUBMED].
59- Farese RVJ, Schambelan M, Hollander H, Stringari S, Jacobson MA. Nephrogenic diabetes insipidus associated with foscarnet treatment of cytomegalovirus retinitis. Ann Intern Med 1990;112:955-6. Back to cited text no. 58 [PUBMED].
60- Greenberg S, Reiser IW, Chou SY. Hyperkalemia with high-dose

trimethoprim-sulphamethaxazole therapy. Am J Kidney Dis 1993;22:603-6. Back to cited text no. 60 [PUBMED].

61- Peter SA. Disorders of serum calcium in acquired immunodeficiency syndrome. J Natl Med Assoc 1992;84:626-8. Back to cited text no. 61 [PUBMED].

62- Kalim S, Szczech LA, Wyatt CM. Acute Kidney Injury in HIV-Infected Patients. Seminars in Nephrology. 2008 11; 28 (6):556-62.

63- Mark AP, Brown E. Electrolyte and Acid-Base Disorders Associated with AIDS: An Etiologic Review. JOURNAL OF GENERAL INTERNAL MEDICINE. 1994 04;9:232-6.

64- Eshiet EM, Jemikalajah DJ, Okogun GRA. Plasma urea and electrolytes profile in different stages of HIV infection in Ekpoma, Nigeria. African Journal of Cellular Pathology. 2015;4:1-5.

65- Ansgar R. Human Immunodeficiency Virus (HIV) and renal function. J. Clin. 2007; 57(2): 15-89.

66- Ross MJ, Klothman PE. HIV-associated nephropathy. Aids. 2004;18: 108999.

67- Onwuliri, VA. Total Bilirubin, Albumin, Electrolytes and Anion Gap in HIV positive patients in Nigeria. J. Med. Sci. 2004; 4(3): 214-20.

68- Berggren, R. and V. Batuman,. HIV-associated renal disorders: recent insights into pathogenesis and treatment. Curr. HIV/AIDS Rep. 2005; 2: 109-15.

# APPENDICES

**Year**

***<u>Enquete form</u>***

**No**

## I. Socio-demographic data

AgeansSex [ ] 1=Male 2=Female

Rësidence

Profession

Ethnic group

Marital status [ ]

1= cëlibataire 2= marie 3= concubinage 4= Veuf 5= divorcë 6= non renseigner

## II. Medical history

HTA [ ] Diabëte [ ] Chronic renal failure on hemodialysis [ ]

Other to be specified

## III. Clinical data

-Reason(s) for hospitalisation :

Diarrhea [ ] Long-term fever [ ] Uncontrollable vomiting [ ] Psychomotor agitation [ ]

Delirium [ ] Chronic cough [ ] Motor neurological deficit [ ]

Others to be specified

-General signs

Etat gen era l Indicede Kamofski% .

Tempërature °C Pulse rate/min

Respiratory ratecycles/minArterial pressuremmHg

Body mass indexkg/$m^2$ (Edemes [ ] i=yes 2=no

-Digestive disorders:

Diarrhoea [ ] vomiting and/or nausea [ ] Anorexia [ ] constipation [ ]

Others to be specified

-State of dehydration

Does it exist? [ ] 1=Yes 2=No

If yes, specify stage [ ] i=Moderate 2= Severe

-Acute malnutrition

Does it exist? [ ] 1=Yes 2=No

If yes, please specify type [ ] 1= Moderate 2= Severe

-Neurological signs :

Irritability [ ] Depression [ ] Disturbance of consciousness [ ] Seizures [ ] Seizures [ ] Other symptoms

Tetany [ ] Midwife's hand [ ] Delirium [ ] Trembling [ ] Other to specify

-Intracranial hypertension :

Cdphaldes [ ] Nausea and/or vomiting [ ] Visual disturbance [ ]

-Muscle signs : fatigability [ ] muscular hypotonia [ ] irregular creur [ ]

-Urinary signs: Polyuria [ ] Oligo-anuria [ ] Macroscopic hematuria [ ] Other to be specified

-Output diagnosis(es) :

Tuberculosis [ ] Non-tuberculous bacterial pneumonia [ ] Cerebral toxoplasmosis [ ] Kaposi's disease [ ] Simple malaria [ ] Severe malaria [ ] Oral candidiasis [ ] Digestive coccidiosis [ ]

Cryptococcosis [ ] Sepsis [ ] 1= pulmonary portal 2= urogenital portal 3= cutaneous portal
Others to be specified
-WHO classification [ ]

**IV. Biological data**

**-Blood count: 1=Normal 2=High 3=Low**

Natremie [ ]
Kaliemie [ ]
Chloremy [ ]
Others to be specified

**- Other tests**

1. **Hemogram** Hemoglobing/dl Hematocrit% Platelets/mm$^3$
2. **Biochemistry**

Creatininepmol/l Creatinine clearanceeml/min Ureemg/l
Glycemiemmol/l Protidemieg/l Albuminemieg/l
Triglyceridemieg/l Other to specify :

3. **Viro-immunology**

HIV type [ ] 1=HIV1 2=HIV2 3=1+2
Viral load (most recent): copies/ml
Absolute CD4 value (most recent) : / mm$^3$
Classification CDC 1993 [ ]

**V-Electrocardiographic data:** ECG [ ] 1=normal 2=rhythm disorders 3=ECG not done

**VI-Therapeutic data**

-ARV treatment [ ] 1=yes 2=no
If yes Duration of ARV treatment :
ARV molecules:- In progress
-Passed schemes
-Related treatments: Sulfamdthoxazole-Trimethoprim [ ], Fluconazole [ ], Amphotdricin B [ ], Aciclovir [ ], Rifampicin Isoniazid Ethambutol Pyrazinamide [ ], Digitalis [ ], Diuretics [ ], Insulin [ ], Mannitol [ ], Others to be specified

**VII-Evolutionary data**

- Becoming **[** ] 1=exeat2=ddces 3=exit without medical advice
-Length of staydays

## Information sheet

**Author:** Dramane SOGOBA
**E-mail:** sogobadramane@yahoo.fr
**Title:** Electrolyte disorders in HIV/AIDS patients hospitalised at the infectious diseases department of the CHU du Point G from January 2011 to December 2016.
**City and year of defence:** Bamako 2017
**Country of origin:** Mali
**Sector of interest :** Nephrology / Infectious diseases
**Place of deposit:** Bibliotheque de la iaculte de mëdecine et d'odontostomatologie, Bamako

**Introduction:** HIV-infected patients, particularly those in the advanced stages of the disease, may be affected by opportunistic diseases. These diseases and their various drug treatments predispose them to develop different kinds of electrolyte disorders. The aim of our work was to analyse these disorders in HIV-infected patients during hospitalisation.

**Materials and methods:** This was a retrospective study conducted in the infectious diseases department of the Point G University Hospital, from 01 January 2011 to 31 December 2016. One hundred and twenty-six HIV-seropositive patients who had a simple blood ionogram during hospitalisation were included.

**Results:** The mean values for natremia were 133.06±12.16 mmol/l, and for kalemia 3.89±1.15 mmol/l, with extremes of 83.00 and 166.00 mmol/l and 1.60 and 9.00 mmol/l respectively. The electrolyte disorders found were hepponatremia (41.2%); livpokalemia (12.7%); hypematremia (7.8%); hyperkalibmia (2.9%) and associated disorders (35.3%).

There was a statistically significant difference between dysnatremia and tuberculosis (p=0.018) and its treatment (p=0.016).

A statistically significant association was also observed between dyskalaemia and cerebral toxoplasmosis (p=0.002); oral candidiasis (p=0.008); diarrhoea (p=0.023); nutritional status (p=0.023); and ARV use (p=0.020). Finally, mortality was related to the level of immunodepression (p=0.012), hydration status (p=0.010) and cerebral toxoplasmosis (p=0.007).

**Conclusion:** Electrolyte disorders are common in patients with HIV/AIDS. Hence the need for regular monitoring of the blood ionogram in these patients during hospitalisation.

**Key words:** HIV, hospitalisation, electrolyte disorders, dysnatremia, dyskaliemia.

**Identification sheet**

**Author:** Dramane SOGOBA
**E-mail:** sogobadramane@yahoo.fr
**Title:** Electrolyte disorders in AIDS patients hospitalized in the department of infectious diseases at the University hospital Point G from January 2011 to December 2016.
**City and Year of defense:** Bamako 2017
**Origin Country:** Mali
**Area of interest:** Nephrology / infectious diseases
**Registration:** Library of the Faculty of Medicine and Dentistry, Bamako

**Introduction:** HIV infected patients; in particular those with advanced disease may be affected by opportunistic diseases. Those diseases and their varied medical treatments predispose them to develop different sort of electrolytes disorders. The aim of this work was to analyze those disorders in HIV infected patients during their hospitalization.

**Material and methods:** it was retrospective study conducted in the department of infectious diseases at the University hospital Point G from 01 january 2011 to 31 december 2016. One hundred and twenty-six HIV positive patients who realized serum sodium, potassium and chloride dosage during their hospitalization have been included there.

**Results:** The mean value was for the serum sodium 133,06±12,16 mmol/l, serum potassium 3,89±1,15 mmol/l with as extreme values respectively 83,00 and 166,00 mmol/l ; 1,60 and 9,00 mmol/l. The electrolyte disorders found were hyponatremia (41,2%) ; hypokaliemia (12,7%) ; hypernatremia (7,8%) ; hyperkaliemia (2,9%) and associated disorders (35,3%).

A significant statistical difference has been observed between dysnatremia and tuberculosis (p=0,018) in part and its treatment (p=0,016) other part.

A significant statistical link has also been found between dyskaliemia and cerebral toxoplasmosis (p=0,002) ; mouth candidiasis (p=0,008) ; diarrhea (p=0,023) ; nutritional status (p=0,023) ; ARV taking (p=0,020). Finally, the mortality was linked to immunosupression level (p=0,012) ; hydratation status (p=0,010) and cerebral toxoplasmosis (p=0,007).

**Conclusion:** The electrolyte disorders are frequent in AIDS patients. The serum electrolyte level must be surveyed regularly in these patients during their hospitalization.

**Key words:** HIV, hospitalization, electrolyte disorders, dysnatremia, dyskaliemia.

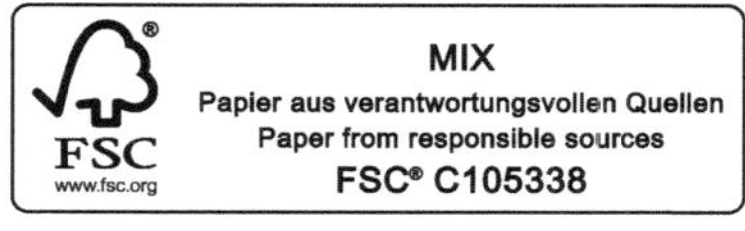


Printed by Books on Demand GmbH, Norderstedt / Germany